# Otosclerosis and Stapedectomy
## Diagnosis, Management, and Complications

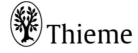 Thieme

# Otosclerosis and Stapedectomy Diagnosis, Management, and Complications

**Christopher de Souza, M.D., F.A.C.S.**
Visiting Assistant Professor in Otolaryngology
State University of New York
Brooklyn, New York
and
Visiting Assistant Professor in Otolaryngology
Louisiana State University Health Science Center
Shreveport, Louisiana
and
Ear, Nose, and Throat and Skull Base Surgeon
Tata Memorial Hospital
Lilavati Hospital
Holy Family Hospital
Holy Spirit Hospital
Mumbai, India

**Michael E. Glasscock, III, M.D., F.A.C.S.**
Clinical Professor Emeritus
Department of Otolaryngology
Vanderbilt University Medical Center
Nashville, Tennessee

## Thieme

New York • Stuttgart

Thieme Medical Publishers, Inc.
333 Seventh Ave.
New York, NY 10001

Assistant Editor: Owen Zurhellen
Consulting Editor: Esther Gumpert
Director, Production and Manufacturing: Anne Vinnicombe
Production Editor: Becky Dille
Marketing Director: Phyllis Gold
Sales Manager: Ross Lumpkin
Chief Financial Officer: Peter van Woerden
President: Brian D. Scanlan
Compositor: Compset, Inc.
Printer: Sheridan Books, Inc.

**Library of Congress Cataloging-in-Publication Data**

De Souza, Chris
  Otosclerosis and stapedectomy: diagnosis, management, and
complications / Christopher de Souza, Michael E. Glasscock III.
      p. ; cm.
Includes bibliographical referencesand index.
  ISBN 1–58890–169–6 TMP : alk. paper—ISBN
  1. Otosclerosis.  2.  Stapedectomy.
  [DNLM: 1. Otosclerosis—surgery. 2. Otosclerosis—diagnosis. 3.
Stapes Surgery. WV 265 D467o 2004] I.  Glasscock, Michael E., 1933– II.
Title.
RF270 .D47 2004
617.8'82—dc22

**Important note:** Medical knowledge is ever-changing. As new research and clinical experience broaden our knowledge, changes in treatment and drug therapy may be required. The authors and editors of the material herein have consulted sources believed to be reliable in their efforts to provide information that is complete and in accord with the standards accepted at the time of publication. However, in the view of the possibility of human error by the authors, editors, or publisher, of the work herein, or changes in medical knowledge, neither the authors, editors, or publisher, nor any other party who has been involved in the preparation of this work, warrants that the information contained herein is in every respect accurate or complete, and they are not responsible for any errors or omissions or for the results obtained from use of such information. Readers are encouraged to confirm the information contained herein with other sources. For example, readers are advised to check the product information sheet included in the package of each drug they plan to administer to be certain that the information contained in this publication is accurate and that changes have not been made in the recommended dose or in the contraindications for administration. This recommendation is of particular importance in connection with new or infrequently used drugs.

Some of the product names, patents, and registered designs referred to in this book are in fact registered trademarks or proprietary names even though specific reference to this fact is not always made in the text. Therefore, the appearance of a name without designation as proprietary is not to be construed as a representation by the publisher that it is in the public domain.

Printed in the United States of America

5 4 3 2 1

TMP ISBN 1–58890–169–6
GTV ISBN 3 13 136051 8

This book is dedicated to Evi Maria, Priyanka, Tara, and Rosemarie.

# Contents

# Foreword

The ankylosis of the stapes was first described by Valsalva[1] in 1735 when he performed an autopsy on a deaf patient. In 1841, Toynbee[2] reported 1659 cases of stapes fixation at autopsy. Politzer was the first to associate stapes ankylosis with a primary disease of the labyrinthine capsule in 1893.[3]

There are many theories on the etiology of otosclerosis that are not in the scope of an introduction. There are numerous sources for this information.[4]

Attempts to improve hearing by attacking stapes fixation in the oval window date back to 1878 when Kessel[5] exposed the middle ear and attempted to mobilize the stapes. Miot[6] reported 200 cases of stapes mobilization with results similar to those reported by Rosen[7] in 1952. It was Lempert[8] who proved that it was possible to operate on the inner ear without producing a sensorineural hearing loss. His one stage fenestration opened the door for the successful stapes surgery that followed. Shea[9] revised the stapedectomy of Blake[10] and Jack,[11] and had the advantage of modern antibiotics and the operating microscope. Shea's great improvement over the earlier surgeons work was his realization that to be successful, the ossicular chain must be reconstructed, after the stapes has been removed. He accomplished this by placing a tissue seal over the open oval window and using a prosthesis from the long process of the incus to the tissue seal.

Over the years, there have been a number of variations on the theme of stapes surgery. Many different prosthesis have been suggested by a variety of otologic surgeons as the best one to use. In recent years, the stapedotomy procedure has produced a great deal of interest.[10] Lasers, both CO2 and argon, have been employed successfully in stapedectomies as well as stapedotomies.[12]

Stapes surgery of either variety is successful in a high percentage of cases regardless of the technique used. Most surgeons report closure of the air-bone gap to within 10dB in over ninety percent of the cases. Dead ears occur somewhere between .5 and 3 percent.[13-15]

What is as important as the surgical skill of the otologist, is the fact that other than the fixation of the stapes, these ears are generally normal in all other aspects. In other words, they have normal Eustachian tube function, middle ear mucosa, and tympanic membranes.

The future always holds surprises. Perhaps in the next few years surgery will be obsolete. With all that is occurring in the field of genetics, gene manipulation may someday be the treatment of choice.

Just think what Valsalva would think if he could walk into a modern operating room and observe a laser-assisted stapedotomy through an observation tube or better still, on a three-dimensional color television screen.

*Michael E. Glasscock III*

# REFERENCES

1. Valsalva AM. *Opera, hoc est, tractatus de aure humana.* Venice; Pitteri: 1735.
2. Toynbee, J. Pathological and surgical observations on the diseases of the ear. *Medico-Chir Tr.* 1841;24:190.
3. Politzer A. Ueber primare Erkrankung der knochernen Labyrinthkapsel. *Ztschr Ohrenh.* 1893;25:309.
4. Shea JJ, Shea PF, McKenna MJ. *Surgery of the Ear*, vol. 5. 2002;519–520.
5. Kessel J. Uber ds Mobilisieren des Stiegbugels durch Ausschneiden des Trommelfelles, Hammers und Amboss bei undurchgangigkeit der Tuba. *Arch Ohrenh.* 1878;13:69.
6. Miot C. De la mobilization de l'etrier. *Rev. Laryng.* 1890;10:49, 83, 145, 200.
7. Rosen S. Palpation of stapes for fixation: preliminary procedure to determine fenestration suitability for otosclerosis. *Arch Otol.* 1952;56:610.
8. Lempert J. Improvement of hearing in cases of otosclerosis: new one-stage surgical technic. *Arch Otolarnygol.* 28:42, 1938
9. Shea JJ Jr. Fenestration of the oval window. *Ann Otol Rhin Laryng.* 1958;67:932.
10. Blake CJ. Middle ear operations. *Tr Am Otol Soc.* 1892;5:2, 306.
11. Jack FL. Further observations on removal of the stapes. *Tr Am Otol Soc.* 1893;5:3, 474.
12. Perkins RC. Laser stapedectomy for otosclerosis. *Laryngoscope.* 1980;90:880.
13. Sheehy JL, House HP. Causes of failure in stapes surgery. *Laryngoscope.* 1962; 73:10–31.
14. Hough JVD. Recent advances in otosclerosis. *Arch Otolaryngol.* 1966;83:379–390.
15. Schuknecht HF. Sensorineural; hearing loss following stapedectomy. *Arch Otolaryngol.* 1962;54:336–347.

# Preface

Stapedectomy still remains one of the most demanding and technical surgeries. There is virtually little room for error and the first surgical effort should be the best effort. In addition the experience garnered by earlier surgeons remains a distant dream for otological surgeons of today. For instance Jean Bernard Causse, a pioneer in this field had performed 25,000 stapedectomies in his lifetime. For today's surgeon this would be next to impossible to accomplish in a single lifetime.

I have been very fortunate to have first trained with Dr. Michael Paparella and then with Dr. Michael Glasscock. Through Dr. Paparella I received a clear insight as to how the otosclerotic process acted on temporal bones. The temporal bone laboratory at the University of Minnesota remains one of the finest in the world and it was there that I received several opportunities to look at the many temporal bones of patients who had suffered from otosclerosis. The microphotographs that appear in this book have been generously supplied by Dr. Paparella from the temporal bone lab at the University of Minnesota. I also had the unique opportunity to see Dr. Paparella operate on patients suffering from otosclerosis. This served to provide me the unique chance to translate histopathologial findings into clinical applications. Mike Paparella has provided many students all over the world a superb understanding not only of otosclerosis but also of many other otological problems. I am among many others who are indebted to him for this unique learning experience. Dr. Marcos Goycoolea, who studied otosclerosis extensively, also influenced me deeply with his observations on otosclerosis. Dr. Goycoolea wrote one of the finest chapters on otosclerosis in the book edited by Dr. Paparella.

Later, I worked with Dr. Michael Glascock in Nashville at Baptist Hospital. This was the turning point in my life. It was there that I saw first hand the vastness of Dr. Glasscock's experience with otosclerosis. I saw virgin stapedectomies, revision stapedectomies, re-revision stapedectomies, and so on. I also saw many patients who were referred by other physicians to Dr. Glasscock for surgery. Many of these had developed complications and were sent to him for treatment. It was here that the complexity of the approach to managing the patient suffering from otosclerosis really became apparent, especially if the patient had undergone unsuccessful surgery elsewhere. Decision making, timing of surgery, which ear to operate on and all the debates that one reads about in textbooks were brought to life in Dr. Glasscock's practice. It was a very edifying experience to have trained with Dr. Glasscock and I will always remain deeply indebted to him for his willingness to share his thoughts, expertise, and experience with all those who were unafraid to approach him. He gave me not only his professional experience but also his warm, deep, and gracious personal friendship. To all his many students Dr. Glasscock will always be a legend. I have a great sense of pride and honor to assist Mike as a coauthor on this book.

I'd also like to thank Dr. C. Gary Jackson who was Mike's partner in Nashville. Gary has a tremendous sense of humor and keen observation. Gary's work was also extensive and we shared many a lively debate. I deeply appreciated everything I learned from Gary's wide experience.

I am deeply appreciative of the team at Thieme. J. Owen Zurhellen, Esther Gumpert, and Becky Dille, who were amazingly efficient, meticulous, and professional. They were also very, very kind.

I'd like to thank Mr. Herman Rodrigues for all his help, time, and expertise that he generously gave to me.

Finally in conclusion it has been my observation that all authors in their books end up thanking their families. I agree and I agree with a lot of certainty. This is so because time spent working on a book means time away from the family. So Mommy has been instrumental in a big way because she has been Mommy and Daddy to the children while Daddy works at being an author.

*Chris de Souza, M.D., F.A.C.S.*
*July 10, 2003*

# Chapter *1*

# The Historical Background of Otosclerosis

Otosclerosis is a disorder that affects the otic capsule exclusively. The term *otosclerosis* is itself actually a misnomer. It is localized otoporosis, not sclerosis of the otic capsule in its active stage. Many authors prefer the term *otospongiosis* because they feel this word more accurately describes the disease in its active phase. For the purposes of convenience, the disease is described as otosclerosis for the rest of this book.

It was Italian anatomist Valsalva who,on a postmortem examination of a deaf patient, described ankylosis of the stapes to the margins of the oval window. English otogist Toynbee noted osseous ankylosis in his dissection of over a thousand temporal bones. It was Politzer who first applied the term *otosclerosis*. He based this on his findings on temporal bones of patients whom he had diagnosed to be suffering from "deafness that had previously been attributed to chronic interstitial middle ear catarrh with secondary stapes ankylosis." Politzer's discovery was confirmed by Bezold and by Siebenmann. In 1912, Siebenmann proposed a change in nomenclature from *otosclerosis* to *otospongiosis*. This change received support from the French otologist Sourdille.

In 1950, Raymond Thomas Carhart, an audiologist, originated the term *air-bone gap*. He reported the notching in bone conduction in the condition of stapedial otosclerosis, notching that has been subsequently known as Carhart's notch. Carhart in 1964, and again in 1966, described audiometric findings that were typical of stapedial and cochlear otosclerosis.

## EVOLUTION OF STAPES SURGERY

In 1878, Kessel described the first successful stapes surgery. The patient, a young man who had been diagnosed as suffering from otosclerosis, had fallen off a wagon and struck his head on the ground. After a brief spell of unconsciousness, the young man found that his sense of hearing had greatly improved. The patient later died of his injuries, and Kessel was able to study his temporal bones. He concluded that the stapes had been mobilized and tried to duplicate this in his surgeries.

Many others attempted to emulate Kessel's work. Boucheron in France reported using techniques similar to that of Kessel. In 1890, Miot reported a series of 200 stapes mobilizations without a single death or labyrinthine complication. All this was done using gaslight and a reflector and local anesthesia.

Blake from Boston in 1892 and Jack in 1893 also reported good results from stapes mobilizations. It was in 1900 at the International Congress of Otolaryngologists in Europe that Politzer and Siebenmann condemned stapes surgery because of its potential to cause meningitis. The result of this public condemnation caused a complete halt to stapes surgery for the next quarter century.

## FENESTRATION OF THE LABYRINTH

In 1916, Holmgren began a long series of operations for stapes ankylosis. He demonstrated that by using careful sterile techniques, the labyrinth could be safely opened. Holmgren's assistant, Nylen, first employed the microscope for ear surgery. Holmgren was not successful, however, in maintaining an open fenestra. In 1924, Sourdille devised a procedure that he termed tympanolabyrithopexy. This two-stage procedure began to give lasting results. Sourdille's success lay in covering the fistula in the horizontal semicircular canal with a very thin skin of the external auditory canal.

Lempert, in 1941, found that extraction of the incus did not cause a reduction in hearing; rather, it provided him with more space to create a wider fenestra over the ampullated end of the lateral semicircular canal. Lempert's was a one-stage technique.

In 1953, Rosen accidentally mobilized the stapes of a patient under local anesthesia. The patient reported that his hearing had suddenly improved. In 1956, Shea reported the first stapedectomy using the operating microscope. Shea sealed the oval window and placed a homograft bone implant between the oval window and the incus; there was an immediate hearing gain. Over time, a conductive hearing loss reappeared because of adhesions. Shea soon replaced that with a Teflon replica of the stapes.

In 1960, Shea inserted a Teflon piston into a small fenestra; thus, stapes surgery was born. Also in that year, Schuknecht used a stainless steel wire prosthesis placed against Gelfoam to seal the oval window.

## REFERENCES

Howard HP. The evolution of otosclerosis surgery. *Otolaryngol Clin North Am.* 1993;26:323–333.

Shambaugh GE. Definition and historical background. In: Wiet RJ, Causse JB, Shambayh GE, Causse JR, eds. *Otosclerosis (Otospongiosis).* American Academy of Otolaryngology—Head and Neck Surgery Foundation; Alexandria, Va; 1991;9–23.

*Chapter 2*

# The Pathology of Otosclerosis

Otosclerosis is a primary and exclusive disease affecting only the otic capsule and the ossicles. It is a localized disorder of bone metabolism of the otic capsule avascular endochondral bone that is characterized by disordered resorption and deposition of bone. Otosclerosis occurs only in the temporal bone (Wang et al 1999).

## ETIOLOGY

The exact etiology of otosclerosis is not known at this time, although many theories have been postulated. None of these theories have been proven to be a definite cause of otosclerosis. Postulated etiologies are hereditary factors, endocrine and metabolic factors, and vascular factors.

Alterations in vascularity (either an increase or a decrease in blood supply) have been postulated by Witmaack (1930), Wolff (1950), and Mendoza and Ruis (1966) to play a role in the etiology of otosclerosis. Intrinsic and extrinsic mechanical stresses as the result of an erect posture were once considered (Mayer 1917) as a cause of otosclerosis, because the petrous pyramid is located at the base of the skull. Because it was located at the base of the skull, it was subjected to mechanical strains exceeding the physiological limits of tolerance, which resulted in defects in the endochondral layer of the bony labyrinth. It was further theorized that the stress factors appeared during the phylogenic and otogenic development due to rotation of the petrous bones at the base of the skull. It was thought that the cochlea moved forward and upward and the vertical semicircular canals backward and downward. Thus, the petrous pyramid has an almost horizontal position in humans versus a vertical position in quadrupeds. This theory was abandoned because otosclerotic changes first appeared in the footplate of the stapes. Fowler (1949) suggested that otosclerosis might be an expression of a general mesenchymal hypoplasia. This was further supported by Ogilvie and Hall (1962), who postulated that otosclerosis was a local manifestation of osteogenesis imperfecta. In recent times viral infections and autoimmune factors have also been postulated to trigger the otosclerotic processes.

Ruedi (1963) demonstrated shunts between the vascular system of the otosclerotic bone and the inner ear, and suggested that venous stasis from these shunts might be responsible for sensorineural hearing loss.

## Clinical Presentation

### Age of Onset

It is difficult to assess the true onset of otosclerosis because the development of histopathologic changes is gradual. Clinical otosclerosis is commonly seen between the ages of 30 and 40 (Nager 1969), with the average age of presentation being 33. DeJuan (1960), comparing the age of onset among various age groups, noted that 28% of cases occurred between ages 18 and 21, 40% presented between ages 21 and 30, and 22% presented between ages 31 and 40. The clinical presentation of otosclerosis is usually that of a conductive hearing loss, which may be unilateral or bilateral. Occasionally it may present as a sensorineural hearing loss. The onset of hearing loss is usually between the fourth and fifth decades, with a higher prevalence in women than men (in the ratio of 2:1). Hearing impairment reaches its maximum in the third decade and then usually remains stable (Glorig and Gallo 1962).

### Prevalence

The prevalence of otosclerosis has been reported as 0.1 to 1.0%, with an average of 0.3% (Gordon, 1989). Autopsy studies (Konigsmark and Gorlin 1976) have found histologic otosclerosis in 5 to 18% of the general population. Jahn and Vernick (1986) stated that 10% of Caucasians develop histologic otosclerosis, and 1% go on to develop clinical otosclerosis. Shambaugh (1961) found that histological otosclerosis was 10 times more common than clinical otosclerosis. Friedmann (1974) and Morrison (1967), however, found the incidence to be approximately 2%. It can therefore be seen that the exact incidence of clinical otosclerosis is not clear and next to impossible to determine. Many authors have noted that in recent years the incidence of patients presenting with otosclerosis has fallen dramatically. The prevalence varies in racial populations, being rare, for example, in African blacks and Asians.

### Race

There is a definite racial predisposition. Otosclerosis is more commonly found in Caucasians. Clinical otosclerosis has been reported to be present in 1% of the population of the United Kingdom, occurring mostly among white females (Hinchcliffe 1961). Guild (1944) reported histologic evidence of otosclerosis in 18.5% of middle-aged white women, 9.7% of adult white men, and only 1% of adult blacks. Cawthorne (1952) found that otosclerosis was more prevalent in fair-haired men than in dark-haired men. The prevalence of otosclerosis is low among Asians (Altmann et al 1967; Nakamura 1968). The prevalence of otosclerosis is low among Japanese (Goto and Omori 1957; Horiguchi 1953; Takahara et al 1959), Chinese, and Indonesians (Nizar 1960). In a comparative study conducted in Hawaii, Joseph and Frazer (1964) found the incidence of otosclerosis to be more prevalent in Caucasians than in Japanese. Rosen and coworkers (1962) did not find clinical cases of otosclerosis in Sudan. Among the Todas in India, however, the prevalence of otosclerosis was estimated at 17%. Kapur and Patt (1966) emphasized the presence of consanguineous marriages, a custom among the

Todas. Consanguinity would then appear to influence the data retrieved. The prevalence of otosclerosis in Native Americans is extremely low across the North American continent (Cambon et al, 1965). Wiet (1979) evaluated a large number of Native Americans and found that only 10 had undergone stapedectomy, of which only three had confirmed otosclerosis, a number representing a minute fraction of the entire population examined. Tato and Tato (1967, 1969) evaluated 5000 Native Americans and found no cases of otosclerosis at all. When there is a racial mixture, however, otosclerosis begins to manifest itself (Goycoolea 1991).

## Gender

Otosclerosis is thought to be more prevalent in women. Schmidt (1933) quoted a female preponderance of 72.5% incidence, whereas Shambaugh (1952) found an incidence of 68% and Cawthorne (1955) an incidence of 67% of women who developed otosclerosis. Because otosclerosis is not a genetically sex-linked characteristic, a ratio of 1:1 would have been expected. However, this has not been found to be true. Endocrinologic factors have been suspected in women. Hueb et al (1991) found a higher incidence of bilateral otosclerosis in women than in men, thus prompting them to believe that women would be more likely to seek medical advice than men. This might possibly account for the apparent gender predisposition.

## OTOSCLEROSIS AND PREGNANCY

Otosclerosis becomes evident during the childbearing years. Most authors report otosclerosis becoming aggravated during pregnancy. Shambaugh (1967) analyzed 475 female patients and reported that 50% did not find any hearing impairment following pregnancies, whereas 8% noticed hearing impairment immediately following pregnancy. In the remaining 42% of patients, hearing loss was associated with pregnancy. Thus, in Shambaugh's series there is a 50% chance of an association of hearing loss following pregnancy. Repeated pregnancies in the same woman, however, did not further worsen hearing. Walsh (1954) found no evidence of a relationship between hearing loss, pregnancy, and otosclerosis. Shambaugh (1967) estimated that the risk of hearing loss to a woman following pregnancy is approximately 1 in 24. Elbrond and Jensen (1979) and Gristwood and Venables (1983) also noted the association of hearing loss following pregnancy. Elbrond and Jensen (1979) studied the hearing threshold of 144 women before and after stapedectomy. The women were between 16 and 40 years old, and all had undergone stapedectomy for otosclerosis. The observation period for the women who became pregnant following stapedectomy was between 4 years and 9 months and 5 years and 8 months. The authors observed that (1) hearing loss became greater in those who became pregnant than in those who did not and (2) the hearing loss became significantly greater in the nonoperated ear of those patients who became pregnant following surgery. It would thus seem that stapedectomy confers some protection from further hearing loss following pregnancy. Although these authors note a correlation between pregnancy and the onset of hearing loss following pregnancy, they are not clear on how this occurs. Morrison (1979) attributed this to increased estrogen levels, which cause fragility of the lysosomal membranes, with the

5

consequent release of enzymes that in turn activate the otosclerotic process. Causse and Causse (1991) postulated that the otosclerotic process is stimulated by the release of increased quantities of estrogen. The increase in estrogen levels causes the lysosomal membranes to become fragile, which in turn leads to the rupture of the membranes with the consequent diffusion of their enzymes, resulting in the destruction of the cochlea and its structures.

## DOES OTOSCLEROSIS PRESENT ONLY AS A CONDUCTIVE HEARING LOSS?

A progressive conductive hearing loss in adults is typical of the way otosclerosis presents (Chole and McKenna 2001). This is due to the fixation of the stapedial footplate along its anterior anulus. On rare occasions, otosclerosis can be associated with sensorineural hearing loss (Schuknecht and Kirchner 1974). This is due to cochlear otosclerosis. It is thought that some individuals may present with cochlear otosclerosis in the absence of a conductive hearing loss.

Temporal bone studies have shown that involvement of the endosteal portion of the cochlea is associated with sensorineural hearing loss and diminished bone conduction hearing thresholds (Ghorayeb and Linthicum, 1978; Hueb et al, 1991). Hyalinization of the spiral ligament adjacent to the otosclerotic foci has been shown to be associated with sensorineural hearing loss (Antoli-Candela et al 1977; Gussen 1975; Hinojosa and Marion 1987).

## HISTOLOGIC OTOSCLEROSIS

Although less than 1% of the population develops clinical otosclerosis, the finding of an otosclerotic focus upon autopsy is much more common. Histologic otosclerosis (Guild 1944) is a disease process without clinical symptoms or manifestations and can only be discovered by routine sectioning of temporal bones (Fig. 2–1) at autopsy. Histologic otosclerosis may be seen as an incidental postmortem finding without causing clinical symptoms. Clinical otosclerosis is otosclerosis at a site where it causes a hearing loss, which may be conductive, sensorineural, or mixed. Histologic otosclerosis has been reported as 8.3% and 11% in large random autopsy series.

Otosclerotic foci can sometimes be seen on high-resolution computed tomography (CT) scans of the temporal bone as areas of hypodensity of the otic capsule or in the vicinity of the oval window (Valvassori 1993). CT scanning, however, is not reliable in detecting otosclerosis, especially when the lesions are sclerotic (Thiers et al 1999). It is possible that future advances in CT imaging and densitometry may be more sensitive in the detection of these lesions. Otosclerotic lesions may also show contrast enhancement on magnetic resonance imaging (Ziyeh et al 1997).

## SIMILAR DISORDERS

Otosclerosis, or otosclerotic-like lesions of the footplate and otic capsule, has been observed in other inherited bone disorders. Otosclerosis is also seen in some patients with osteogenesis imperfecta who commonly develop conductive hearing loss. The lesions in the temporal bone appear similar to

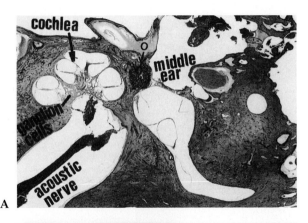

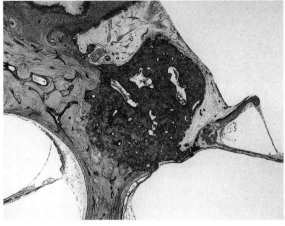

**Figure 2–1** **(A)** Photomicrograph of a human temporal bone with histologic otosclerosis (O). This focus lies anterior to the oval window and has not resulted in any symptoms. This is an incidental finding on autopsy, discovered accidentally, and is termed *histologic otosclerosis*. **(B)** Magnified view of the same human temporal bone section demonstrating histologic otosclerosis.

those of otosclerosis (Nager 1988), although some patients have lesions consisting of diminished calcification and microfractures. The bony lesions of Paget's disease in the otic capsule may appear similar to otosclerosis, although their distribution within the temporal bone is distinct (Fig. 2–2). Large multinucleate osteoclasts are much more prominent in Paget's disease than in otosclerosis. It must be stated that the conductive hearing losses sometimes associated with Paget's disease are not due to ossicular lesions, but may be due to the loss of mineral density in the otic capsule (Khetarpal and Schuknecht 1990). Paget's disease of the bone, like otosclerosis, is a disorder of localized bone remodeling, with osteoclastic resorption followed by compensatory increases in bone formation. Paget's disease affects localized regions of the skeleton while sparing others; however, unlike otosclerosis, it is not restricted to the temporal bone. Thirty percent of those suffering from Paget's have a family history of the disease, causing speculation about a genetic basis of this disease. There is recent evidence from linkage studies

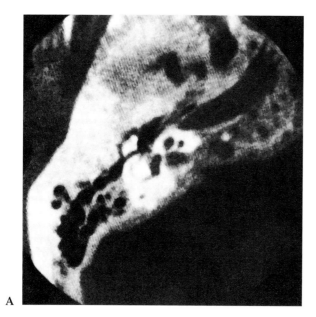

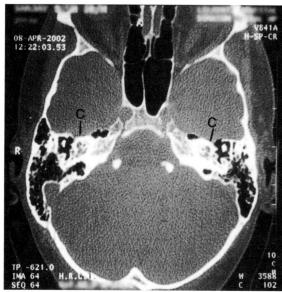

**Figure 2–2** Computed tomography (CT) scan **(A)** of a patient suffering from Paget's disease. Compare this with a CT scan **(B)** of a patient suffering from cochlear otosclerosis. The cochlea in **(A)** is normal, but the cochlea **(C)** in **(B)** is lucent.

that chromosome 18 carries a predisposition gene for Paget's disease (Leach et al 1999). In addition, there is compelling evidence of a viral etiology in Paget's disease (Mills et al 1994). Paget's disease may cause conductive and/or sensorineural hearing loss by involvement of the otic capsule and ossicles. Otosclerotic-like changes have also been described in Camurati-Engelmann disease (CED) (Chole and McKenna 2001). CED, also known as progressive diaphyseal dysplasia, is a rare disorder of rapid bone turnover, diaphyseal hyperostosis, and muscle hypoplasia. Affected individuals commonly experience mixed hearing loss and vertigo. Radiologically, lesions similar to otic capsule otosclerosis have been seen (Hanson and Parnes 1995; Huygen et al 1996).

## SITES OF INVOLVEMENT

Otosclerotic foci are commonly found in front of the oval window. This location has been reported in 80 to 90% of temporal bones with otosclerosis (Guild 1944). The second most common site is the round window (Fig. 2–3). Very rarely will the round window be occluded by otosclerosis, with complete obliteration of the round window accounting for 6% of temporal bones examined (Hueb et al 1991). Reports of round window involvement range from 30 to 50% (Guild 1944; Nylen 1949). It was also noted, however, that despite being very close to the round window, otosclerotic focus merged in approximately 12% of cases (Nager 1969). The surgical findings of extensive otosclerosis obliterating the round window have been reported to be approximately 1%. Shea and Farrior (1987) reported this finding in 30,000 patients who had undergone stapedectomy. Schuknecht and Barber (1985) reported involvement of the round window in 30% of cases of clinical otosclerosis and 17% of temporal bones of histologic otosclerosis. Other sites that were involved were the apical medial wall of the cochlea, posterior to the oval window, the posterior internal auditory canal, the cochlea aqueduct, and the semicircular canals. In the same report, involvement anterior to the oval window as the only focus was seen in 51% of cases of clinical otosclerosis. Involvement of the malleus and incus, though uncommon, can cause fixation of the head of the malleus in the attic.

Otosclerosis usually affects both temporal bones symmetrically. Nylen (1949) found that 70 to 80% of cases were involved bilaterally and were

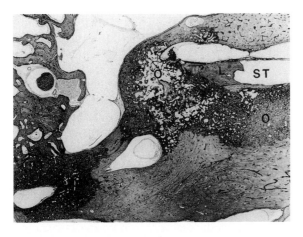

**Figure 2–3** Otosclerotic focus (O) at the round window. New bone formation (L) has replaced the round window. ST = scala tympani.

symmetrical in the areas of involvement. Nagen (1947) found histologically unilateral otosclerosis in 10% of temporal bones.

## ANATOMY OF THE OTIC CAPSULE

Cartilage persists throughout life in certain parts of the otic capsule. Bast and Anson (1949) described seven regions where cartilage has been noted: (1) fissula ante fenestram, (2) fossula post fenestram, (3) intracochlear area (endochondral layer), (4) cochlear area (round window), (5) semicircular canals, (6) petrosquamous suture, and (7) base of the styloid process.

The otic capsule consists of three layers: the endochondral, the periosteal, and the endosteal. The endochondral layer is located lateral to the endosteal layer and medial to the periosteal layer. It contains areas of calcified cartilaginous matrix, and occasionally cartilage cells remain. The calcified areas have capillary buds. Osteoblasts deposit bone in the lacunae, forming small bony globules, or globuli ossei. The primitive perichondrium (Bast and Anson 1949) becomes the periosteum or the periosteal layer.

The fissula ante fenestram is located anterior to the oval window and is the most common site for otosclerosis. In 70 to 90% of cases, otosclerotic lesions may replace the fissula ante fenestram (Nager 1969). The fissula ante fenestram forms a fibrous connection between the periotic tissues and the tissues of the middle ear. The fissula reduces in size when a new secondary cartilage is produced from the perichondrium.

The fossula post fenestram is an evagination of the periotic tissue into the cartilaginous capsule just posterior to the oval window. The fossula is also commonly involved by otosclerotic lesions.

## HISTOPATHOLOGY

### Light Microscopy

Otosclerosis is a localized bone remodeling process that occurs in the otic capsule. The otic capsule and the ossicles arise from cartilaginous anlage by endochondral calcification. The calcification process is completed by 1 year of age. Once calcified, the otic capsule exhibits little remodeling. There is evidence that a low level of bone remodeling occurs within the otic capsule, as seen on fluorochrome labeling experiments in a number of mammals, including humans. It is of deep interest that remodeling of the otic capsule is at a very low level as compared with other parts of the skeleton. Osteoblastic and osteoclastic activity, normally associated with bone turnover, is rarely seen in the adult otic capsule. The otic capsule contains small regions of immature cartilaginous tissue called globuli interossei, which may be the loci of the earliest lesions of otosclerosis.

Early phases are characterized by resorption of bone around blood vessels, with an increase in space and size around vascular channels (Fig. 2–4). Vascular spaces become wider. There is a decalcifying process related to the lacunar system and osteophytes. The initial stages are characterized by diffuse or patchy demineralization that coincides with preotosclerotic lesions in light microscopy (Lim 1970; Lim and Saunders 1977). The blood vessels in the marrow spaces are increased and become dilated. If the active focus reaches the periosteal surface of the promontory, dilated blood vessels may

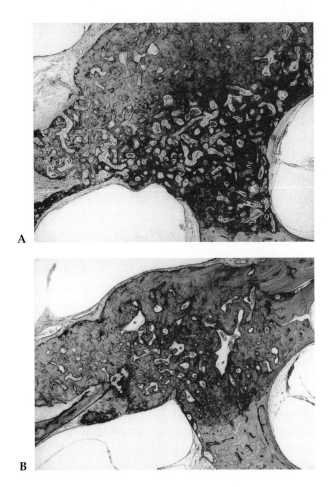

**Figure 2–4** **(A)** Photomicrograph of active otosclerosis as indicated by increased vascular spaces. **(B)** Photomicrograph of human temporal bone depicting otosclerotic focus slowly becoming inactive.

cause a red-pink glow that can be seen through the tympanic membrane, a glow known as Schwartze's sign. Schwartze's sign represents vascular shunts between vessels in the otosclerotic focus and the submucosal vessels of the promontory.

Otosclerotic foci may appear as dense mineralized bone (sclerotic bone) or as active, well-vascularized bone (spongiotic bone). One of the earliest manifestations of otosclerosis is the "blue mantle" within the otic capsule. Blue mantles are basophilic staining regions that are seen in the otic capsule near regions of otosclerosis in temporal bones that have been stained with hemotoxylin and eosin (Manasse 1922; Weber 1933). Blue mantles (of Manasse) are nonspecific histologic changes characterized by plexus-like projections. They are formed by resorptive spaces in the otic capsule surrounding vascular spaces that stain markedly with the blue of hemotoxylin and have a mantle-like appearance; hence the name. They may be the earliest histologic evidence of otosclerosis and may occur in isolation. These regions probably represent bone that has been remodeled recently. This basophilic bone may

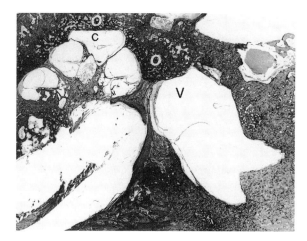

**Figure 2–5** Photomicrograph of advanced otosclerotic (O) focus deforming the cochlea (C) and vestibule (V).

be new bone that has been deposited in a Howship's lacuna after osteoclastic resorption in the vicinity of a blood vessel or merely a change in the staining pattern of bone adjacent to the bone-lining cells of vascular spaces.

Otosclerotic remodeling distorts the contours of the labyrinth and the ossicles (Fig. 2–5). Otosclerotic bone replaces normal endochondral bone and can become exophytic and extend into the middle ear and into the perilymphatic spaces. Within an active otosclerotic focus, osteoclasts and osteoblasts can be seen. The otosclerotic focus is made up of bone formation by osteoblasts, bone destruction by osteoclasts, vascular proliferation, and a stroma of fibroblasts and histiocytes.

The most common location of an otosclerotic focus is that area of the otic capsule anterior to the stapedial footplate (the region of the fissula ante fenestram) (Schuknecht and Barber, 1985). Otosclerotic foci have been found only in the temporal bone. Involvement of the otic capsule without involvement of the ossicles is rare.

## Electron Microscopy

Light and electron microscopy studies reveal that the majority of cells present within active otosclerotic lesions are mononuclear and appear to represent osteoblasts and osteoclast precursors. The other common cells found in active lesions are histiocytes and tissue macrophages. There is a distinct absence of acute inflammatory cells. In active lesions, the most common cell type seen is osteoclasts. An extremely common feature seen in active lesions is the frequent disruption of osteoblasts with marked dilatation of the endoplasmic reticulum. Less active lesions display new woven bone formation with hypercellularity, often with more than two cells situated within a single lacuna. The extracellular matrix consists of disoriented collagen fibrils with a normal banding pattern. Of particular significance is the presence of undulating filamentous structures within the dilated endoplasmic reticulum, cytosol, and occasional nuclei of osteoblasts and preosteoblasts in active lesions. They are morphologically similar to measles virus nucleocapsid and the nucleocapsid structures seen in subacute sclerosing panencephalitis. Unlike Paget's disease, viral-like structures have not been observed within the osteoclasts or osteoclast nuclei (McKenna 1996; McKenna and Mills 1990).

## OTOSCLEROSIS: A DISEASE OF ALTERED LOCALIZED BONE REMODELING

In otosclerosis, endochondral bone of the otic capsule is resorbed by osteoclasts, and new bone is deposited by osteoblasts. Within the normal otic capsule, osteoclastic and osteoblastic activity has never been demonstrated. Thus, in otosclerosis, the result is a localized region of poorly organized bone that does not respect the normal contours of the otic capsule.

In the bony skeleton, bone grows and remodels by the action of osteoblasts and osteoclasts. Although other cells, such as osteophytes and bone-lining cells, contribute to calcium flux on bone surfaces, bone remodeling is a process that basically occurs only by the action of osteoclasts and osteoblasts. Activation of osteoclastic activity is always associated with osteoblastic activity. This synergistic activity leads to constant bone remodeling and results in old haversian systems being resorbed and new ones being formed. This occurs throughout the entire bony skeleton with the exception of the otic capsule. After the endochondral bone ossification in early life, osteoclasts and osteoblasts are not seen in the otic capsule.

## GENETICS OF OTOSCLEROSIS

Otosclerosis has long been believed to have a genetic factor. Toynbee (1861) first wrote about the hereditary nature of otosclerosis. Most genetic studies on families with otosclerosis support a pattern of autosomal dominant transmission with incomplete penetrance (Causse and Causse 1984; Larson 1960) (Fig. 2–6). There is growing evidence that suggests that otosclerosis may be a heterogenetic disease, with the typical clinical phenotype arising from more than one possible genetic defect (Ben Arab et al 1993). Morrison and Bundey (1970) demonstrated that 43% of those carrying the abnormal allele develop clinical otosclerosis, and the remaining 57% develop histologic otosclerosis. These 57% are also able to transmit the disease. Causse and Causse (1980) and Causse and Causse (1984), analyzing data from 614 families with 1465 affected members, also found approximately the same findings. Studies involving three to five generations of persons suffering from otosclerosis have been published (Davenport et al 1933; Gregoriadis et al 1982). Mendelowitz and Hirschorn (1976) studied the pedigree of a family and went back six generations. They reported that the mode of inheritance was polygenic and multifactorial, and they found that individuals within the family had an increased risk of having children who developed otosclerosis that manifested itself early and with a severe degree of hearing loss. Those who married outside the family were still exposed to a higher incidence of having children who would develop symptoms related to otosclerosis, although the risks were decreased as compared with the risks if they had married within the family. All point strongly to a genetic inheritance.

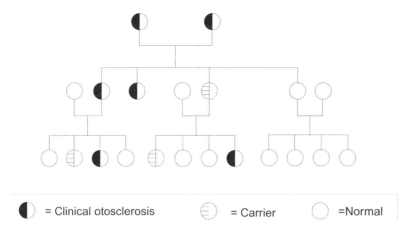

**(●)** = Clinical otosclerosis     **(◒)** = Carrier     **(○)** =Normal

**Figure 2–6**  Chart demonstrating genetic pattern of inheritance of otosclerosis. *(Adapted from Beales, PH.* Otosclerosis. *Bristol: John Wright and Sons; 1981. Used with permission.)*

Evidence that supports a genetic basis comes from studies on monozygotic twins, in which evidence of otosclerosis was found in nearly all the cases (Fowler 1966). In a study of monozygotic twins, Wayoff and colleagues (1979) stressed the hereditary nature of otosclerosis. Ruedi (1963) postulated a monohybrid autosomal inheritance with a penetrance of the gene in a percentage ranging from 25 to 45%. Gapany-Gapanavicius (1975) thought that there was autosomal dominant transmission with incomplete penetrance and variable expressivity. Chobaut and colleagues (1979) reported on the human leukocyte antigen (HLA) system in relation to this disease and found a repitition of B8 antigen and otosclerosis in different races. Gregoriadis et al (1982) found a significantly increased frequency of $A_{11}$, $B_{14}$, and $B_{w35}$ antigens These data give support to the theory that otosclerosis is a hereditary disorder having an autosomal dominant inheritance with approximately 40% penetrance of genes. Linkage studies between otosclerosis and the ABO M:N and Rh blood groups and half the globulin genotypes have failed to demonstrate evidence of linkage. In another study (Singhal et al 1999), 100 patients suffering from otosclerosis were matched with 100 normal controls, and all underwent HLA typing as determined by microlymphocytotoxic assay. The frequencies of the HLA antigens were compared between the otosclerotic patients and the controls. Their findings revealed that patients suffering from otosclerosis had significantly higher levels of HLA-A3 (relative risk [RR] 2.8) HLA-A9 (RR 5.34), HLA-A11 (RR 3.14), and HLA-B13 (RR 4.26). Levels of HLA-A9 and HLA-A11 were significantly higher in male patients, whereas levels of HLA-A3 were significantly higher in female patients. In the 30 patients who had a family history of otosclerosis, HLA-A9 and HLA-A11 levels were still higher. HLA-A1 levels were significantly lower in the otosclerotic patients than they were in the controls (RR 0.38). Chromosomal studies in otosclerosis have demonstrated normal karyotypes (Nitze 1967). This is expected because autosomal transmission is not related to chromosomal abnormalities.

Recently, analysis of a large family from India with a presumptive diagnosis of otosclerosis revealed linkage to a region of chromosome 15q

(Tomek et al 1998). The investigators suggested that the gene for aggrecan, an extracellular matrix protein found predominantly in cartilage, may be a possible candidate gene. Other families have been examined specifically for evidence of linkage to this region, however, and no evidence supporting this theory was found. This again supports the concept of a heterogenetic disorder. Thalmann and colleagues (1987) detected possible alterations in collagenous proteins in otosclerotic tissues. There is recent evidence to suggest that in a small number of cases otosclerosis may be related to gene defects in COL1A1 gene, one of the genes that code for type I collagen, the major collagen component of bone. Analysis has revealed an association between the COL1A1 allelic expression in cultured fibroblasts from individuals with clinical otosclerosis that is either familial or sporadic. Analysis of COL1A1 allelic expression in cultured fibroblasts from individuals with clinical otosclerosis has shown that in a small percentage of cases, ranging from 10 to 20%, one of the COL1A1 alleles is expressed in extremely low reiteration. This is similar to that which is seen in many cases of mild (type I) osteogenesis imperfecta. This suggests that in a small percentage of cases, the underlying genetic mechanism may be very similar to that of osteogenesis imperfecta (McKenna et al 1998). The hearing loss that occurs in persons with type I osteogenesis imperfecta occurs almost exclusively in association with COL1A1 defects and is seen in 50% of affected persons. It shares the same autosomal dominant inheritance with incomplete penetration, as seen with otosclerosis.

Mazzoli, Rosignoli, and Martini (2001) examined sporadic and familial (hereditary) patients suffering from otosclerosis, and reported that in sporadic cases of otosclerosis a genetic cause cannot be excluded because of the possibility of a different mode of inheritance, new mutations, or the absence of expression in family members. They also stated that environmental factors may be responsible for the high degree of variability between families.

## THE ROLE OF MEASLES VIRUS IN OTOSCLEROSIS

There has been increasing evidence that a paramyxovirus may likely be the cause of Paget's disease of the bone. Paget's disease of the bone and otosclerosis are similar pathologies. This in turn has led researchers to look for evidence of a similar etiology for otosclerosis. An increasing body of evidence indicates that the measles virus is a possible etiologic agent in the cause of otosclerosis. The evidence includes transmission electron microscopy, which has demonstrated measles-like structures within active otosclerotic foci. Other evidence includes immunohistochemical evidence of measles antigen in active foci, reverse transcription polymerase chain reaction amplification of measles ribonucleic acid (RNA) from otosclerotic lesions recovered from fresh and stored tissue samples (McKenna and Mills 1989). Additional evidence includes elevated levels of immunoglobulin G (IgG) specific for measles virus antigens in the perilymph of patients suffering from otosclerosis. This was not found in the control group of patients (Niedermeyer and Arnold 1995).

The results of this study suggest that a persistent measles virus infection together with an underlying hereditary predisposition may lead to the development of clinical otosclerosis. This would help explain the sporadic nature of the disease as well as the observed incomplete penetrance of the phenotype. McKenna and colleagues (1998) suggested that the initial otosclerotic lesion may be initiated by measles infection of the globuli interossei, which can account for the sole predilection of the temporal bone. The establishment of persistent infection may be related to the relatively quiescent metabolic state or terminal differentiation of the osteocytes or chondrocytes within the globuli interossei, which results in restricted expression of the measles genome with little or no expression of late viral genes critical for complete viral assembly and escape (Schneider-Schaulies et al 1993). Infected cells produce factors that destabilize the extracellular matrix and lead to activation of the remodeling process. The progression and extension of the abnormal remodeling process are dependent upon an underlying genetic defect in collagen metabolism. There may be multiple different mutations within the COL1A1 gene and in other genes within the collagen metabolism pathway that result in the generation of an unstable extracellular matrix with a high propensity for remodeling. Although multiple different mutations in COL1A1 may result in null expression of the mutant alleles, the downstream effect on other related factors that are critical determinants in the remodeling process may vary among mutations and produce a varied spectrum in clinical and histologic severity. These are new and interesting theories. Additional studies, however, will be required to establish which loci and genes are related to the development of otosclerosis. Furthermore, to substantiate the viral cause of otosclerosis, the virus will need to be isolated from the otosclerotic tissue.

## THE ROLE OF AUTOIMMUNITY IN OTOSCLEROSIS

It was Chevance, Jorgensen, and Causse (1969) who postulated that otosclerosis is a self-maintaining process that is initiated from one or more numerous embryonic cartilaginous remnants that are scattered throughout the endochondral layer of the unstable otic capsule. Bretlau (1973) suggested the possibility of an autoimmune reaction in the unstable cartilage of the otic capsule. Petrovic et al (1985) reported that otosclerosis is indeed an autoimmune disease; they believed that the cellular immune system plays a role in the pathogenesis of otosclerosis. Schiff and Yoo (1985) concluded that otosclerosis could be made to develop locally as a response to inflammation. Huang, Yi, and Abramson (1986) agreed with these findings. Yoo and colleagues (1982) first reported increased type II collagen antibodies in patients suffering from otosclerosis. On the other hand, Sorenson et al (1988) and Lolov et al (1998) found no difference in otosclerotic patients compared with controls. In other later reports, Joliat and colleagues (1992) and Bujia et al (1994) found significantly elevated levels of antibodies to types II and IX in otosclerotic patients compared with controls. Yoo et al (1983) suggested that type II collagen immunity induced in rats leads to bone lesions similar to those seen in otosclerosis, although in a separate and identical study, Harris et al (1986) found no such lesions.

Causse and Causse (1991) believed that a humoral rather than a cellular autoimmune process plays an important role in the pathogenesis of otosclerosis. The stimulation of mononuclear phagocytes by the complement system via the IgG triggers the enzymatic cascade with its consequent destructive process. The authors further believed that an immune process triggering the enzymatic cycle in otosclerosis lies in the possibility of an antigen-antibody reaction in which the embryonic cartilaginous remnants primarily located in the fissula ante fenestram act as an autoantigen (Causse et al 1977). They found it reasonable to believe that the immune mechanism in human otosclerosis is a self-maintaining process. The embryonic cartilaginous remnants located in the endochondral layer of the otic capsule are the major source of type II collagen and therefore the site of the action of the anti–type II collagen antibodies.

Causse and colleagues (1982) evaluated trypsin, alpha$_1$-antitrypsin, and alpha$_2$-macroglobulin levels in 811 samples of perilymph. They found that alpha$_2$-macroglobulin appeared to have a synergistic relationship with alpha$_1$-antitrypsin in the balance with trypsin. They also found the interaction significant because in otosclerosis, the alpha$_1$-antitrypsin values are low. The hydrolytic enzymes and the relatively avascular metabolic isolation of the otic capsule make the disturbance in the trypsin-antitrypsin equilibrium possible. A disturbance in this equilibrium favors tryptic activity. This in turn leads to an increase in trypsin levels, which in turn damages hair cells. The first phase in bone lysis results in the second pseudohaversian bone-rebuilding phase. When the enzymes cause only bone rebuilding because of the second pseudohaversian phase following the lytic process, conductive deafness occurs as a result of stapedial fixation. Sensorineural hearing loss occurs when the enzymes spread into the labyrinthine fluids either by perfusion or through the canaliculi. The balance between trypsin and alpha$_1$-antitrypsin and other protease inhibitors is not the only mechanism involved in otosclerosis. Other enzymes, such as collagenase, alpha chymotrypsin, phosphatic acid, ribonuclease, and lactate dehydrogenase, as well as cathepsin B, have been found in the perilymph of otosclerotic patients.

## ANIMAL MODELS

No convincing animal models for otosclerosis exist. The LP/J mouse develops abnormal bony lesions in the ossicles and otic capsule that are similar grossly and histologically to otosclerosis that is seen in humans. This observation is the first known occurrence of spontaneous otosclerosis-like lesions in animals. These are accompanied, however, by an inflammatory reaction as the lesions advance. The incisor-absent rat also develops otic capsule remodeling. The remodeling process is not limited to the temporal bone.

Biochemical and tissue cultures of bone cells from otosclerotic bones have allowed a better understanding of the molecular basis of this disorder. Clinical and experimental immunological methods help postulate that type I and/or type III immune responses are underlying mechanisms for the pathogenesis of otosclerosis. Better animal models in the future may help us to understand how otosclerosis occurs.

## REFERENCES

Altmann F, Glassgold A, MacDuff JP. The incidence of otosclerosis as related to race and sex. *Ann Otolaryngol.* 1967;76:377–381.

Antoli–Candela F, McGill T, Peron D. Histopathological observations on the cochlear changes in otosclerosis. *Ann Otol, Rhinol Laryngol.* 1977;86:813–820.

Bast H, Anson BJ. *The Temporal Bone and the Ear.* Springfield, IL: Charles C. Thomas; 1949.

Ben Arab S, Bonaiti–Pellie C, Belkahia A. A genetic study of otosclerosis in a population living in the north of Tunisia. *Ann Genetics*. 1993;36:111–116.

Bretlau P. *Otosklerose: histopathologiske under sogelser afdet otosklerotiske focus*. Kobenhaven, Aarhus, Odense; 1973.

Bujia J, Alsalameh S, Jerez R, et al. Antibodies to the minor cartilage collagen type IX in otosclerosis. *Am J Otology*. 1994;15:222–224.

Cambon K, Galbraith JD, Kong G. Middle ear disease in Indians of the Mount Currie reservation, British Columbia. *Canada Med Assoc J*. 1965;92:1301–1305.

Causse JR, Causse JB. L'otospongiose, maladie familiale: sa détection préecoce, son traitement médical. *Ann Otol, Rhinol Laryngol*. 1980;97:325–351.

Causse JR, Causse JB. Otospongiosis as a genetic disease: Early detection, medical management and prevention. *Am J Otology*. 1984;5:211–223.

Causse JR, Causse JB. Pathology. In: Wiet RJ, Causse JB, Shambaugh GE, Causse JR, eds. *Otosclerosis*. American Academy of Otolaryngology/Head and Neck Surgery Foundation; Washington D.C., 1991:30–48.

Causse JR, Chevance LG, Bretlau P, et al. Enzymatic concept of otospongiosis and cochlear otospongiosis. *Clinical Otolaryngology*. 1977;2:23–32.

Causse JR, Urile J, Berges J, et al. The enzymatic mechanism of the otospongiotic disease and NaF action on the enzymatic balance. *Am J Otology*. 1982;3:197–214.

Cawthorne T. Otosclerosis. In: Scott Brown HG, ed. *Diseases of the Ear, Nose and Throat*. London: Butterworth; 1952:29–53.

Cawthorne T. Otosclerosis. *J Laryngol Otology*. 1955;69:437.

Chevance LG, Jorgensen MB, Causse JR. L'otospongiose comme maladie lysosomale. *Proceedings of the Ninth International Congress of Mexico*; 1969:81–86.

Chobaut JC, Bertrand D, Raffoux C, et al. HLA antigens in otosclerosis. *Am J Otology*. 1979;3:241–242.

Chole RS, McKenna M. Pathophysiology of otoscleroosis. *Am J Otolaryngol Neurotol*. 2001;22:249–257.

Davenport CB, Milles BL, Flink LB. The genetic factor in otosclerosis. *Arch Otolaryngol*. 1933;17:135.

DeJuan P. Consideraciones sobre la otosclerosis. *Acta Otolaryngol Iber Am*. 1960;11(5):389–416.

Elbrond O, Jensen KJ. Otosclerosis and pregnancy: A study of the influence of pregnancy on the hearing threshold before and after stapedectomy. *Clin Otolaryngology*. 1979;4:259–266.

Fowler EP. Otosclerosis in identical twins. *Ann Otolaryngology*. 1949;56:368.

Fowler EP. Otosclerosis in identical twins: A study of 40 pairs. *Arch Otolaryngol*. 1966;83:324–328.

Friedmann I. Otosclerosis. In: *Pathology of the Ear*. Oxford: Blackwell; 1974:247.

Gapany–Gapanavicius B. *Otosclerosis: Genetics and Surgical Rehabilitation*. New York: John Wiley and Sons; 1975:177–178.

Ghorayeb BY, Linthicum FH. Otosclerotic inner ear syndrome. *Ann Otol, Rhinol, and Laryngol*. 1978;87:85–90.

Glorig A, Gallo R. Comments on sensorineural hearing loss in otosclerosis. In: Schuknecht HF, ed. *Otosclerosis*. Boston: Little, Brown; 1962:63–78.

Gordon MA. The genetics of otosclerosis: A review. *Am J Otology*. 1989;10:426–438.

Goto H, Omori YL. Otosclerosis in Japan. *Nagoya J Med Sci*. 1957;19:147.

Goycoolea MV. Otosclerosis. In:. Paparella MM, Shumrick DA, Gluckman JL, Meyerhof WL, eds. *Otolaryngology*. Vol 2. 3rd ed. Philadelphia: WB Saunders; 1991:1489–1512.

Gregoriadis S, Zervas J, Varletzidis E, Toubis M, et al. HLA antigens and otosclerosis: A possible new genetic factor. *Arch Otolaryngol*. 1982;108:769–771.

Gristwood RE, Venables WN. Pregnancy and otosclerosis. *Clin Otolaryngol*. 1983;8:205–210.

Guild SR. Histologic otosclerosis. *Ann Otol, Rhinol Laryngol*. 1944;53:246–266.

Gussen R. Labyrinthine otosclerosis and sensorineural deafness: Pathologic findings of the spiral ligament. *Arch Otolaryngol*. 1975;101:438–440.

Hanson W, Parnes LS. Vestibular nerve compression in Camurati–Engelmann disease. *Ann Otol, Rhinol Laryngol*. 1995;104:823–825.

Harris JP, Woolf NK, Ryan AF. A reexamination of experimental type II collagen autoimmunity: Middle and inner ear morphology and function. *Ann Otol, Rhinol Laryngol*. 1986;95:176–180.

Hinchcliffe R. Otosclerosis. *Br Med J*. 1961;15:128–130.

Hinojosa R, Marion M. Otosclerosis and sensorineural hearing loss: A histopathologic study. *Am J Otolaryngol*. 1987;8:296–307.

Horiguchi S. Otosclerosis. *J Pap Oto Rhinol Laryngol*. 1953;56:995–998.

Huang CE, Yi Z, Abramson M. Type II collagen induced otospongiosis like lesions in rats. *Otolaryngol Head Neck Surg*. 1986;7:258–266.

Hueb MM, Goycoolea MV, Paparella MM. Otosclerosis: The University of Minnesota temporal bone collection. *Otolaryngol, Head Neck Surg*. 1991;105:396–405.

Huygen PL, Cremers CW, Verhagen WI, et al. Camurati–Engelmann disease presenting as "juvenile otosclerosis." *Intl J Ped Otorhinolaryngol*. 1996;37:129–141.

Jahn AF, Vernick D. Otosclerosis: Diagnosis and treatment. SIPAC. American Academy of Otolaryngology–Head and Neck Surgery; 1986:12–20.

Joliat T, Seyer J, Bernstein J, et al. Antibodies to a 30 kilodalton cochlear protein and type II and IX collagens in the serum of patients with inner ear diseases. *Ann Otol, Rhinol Laryngol*. 1992;101:1000–1006.

Joseph RB, Frazer JP. Otosclerosis incidence in Caucasians and Japanese. *Arch Otolaryngol*. 1964;80:257–260.

Kapur YP, Patt AJ. Otosclerosis in south India. *Acta Otolaryngol*. 1966;61:353–355.

Khetarpal U, Schuknecht HF. In search of pathologic correlates for hearing loss and vertigo in Paget's disease: A clinical and histopathologic study of 26 temporal bones. *Ann Otol, Rhinol Laryngol*. 1990;145:1–16.

Konigsmark BW, Gorlin RJ. *Genetic and Metabolic Deafness*. Philadelphia: WB Saunders; 1976.

Larson A. Otosclerosis: A genetic and clinical study. *Acta Otolaryngol*. 1960;154:1–86.

Leach RJ, Singer FR, Cody JD, et al. Variable disease severity associated with a Paget's disease predisposition gene. *J Bone Mineral Res*. 1999;14:17–20.

Lim DJ. A scanning electron microscope investigation on otosclerotic stapes. *Ann Otol, Rhinol Laryngol*. 1970;79:780–784.

Lim DJ, Saunders WH. Otosclerotic stapes: Morphological and microchemical correlates. *Ann Otol, Rhinol Laryngol*. 1977;86:525–530.

Lolov SR, Edrev GE, Kyurchiev SD, et al. Elevated autoantibodies in sera from otosclerotic patients are related to the disease duration. *Acta Otolaryngol*. 1998;118:375–380.

Manasse P. Neue unterschungen zur otosklerosenfrage. *Z Ohrenheilk*. 1922;82:76–96.

Mayer O. *Unterschusuchugen über die Otosklerose*. Vienna and Leipzig: Alfred Holder; 1917:80.

Mazzoli M, Rosignoli M, Martini A. Otosclerosis: Are familial and isolated cases different disorders? *J Audiological Med*. 2001;10:1:49–59.

McKenna MJ. Polymerase chain reaction amplification of a measles virus sequence from human temporal bone sections with active otosclerosis. *Am J Otolaryngol*. 1996;17:827–830.

McKenna MJ, Kristiansen AG, Bartley ML, et al. Association of COL1A1 and otosclerosis: Evidence for a shared genetic etiology with mild ostogenesis imperfecta. *Am J Otolaryngol*. 1998;19:604–610.

McKenna MJ, Mills BG. Immunohistochemical evidence of measles virus antigens in active otosclerosis. *Otolaryngol Head Neck Surg*. 1989;101:415–421.

McKenna MJ, Mills BG. Ultrastructural and immunohistochemical evidence of measles virus in active otosclerosis. *Acta Otolaryngol*. 1990; 470(suppl):130–140.

Mendelowitz JC, Hirschorn K. Polygenic inheritance of otosclerosis. *Ann Otol, Rhinol Laryngol*. 1976;85:281–285.

Mendoza D, Ruis M. Histology of the endochondral layer of the human otic capsule. *Acta Otolaryngol*. 1966;62:93.

Mills BG, Frausto A, Singer FR, et al. Multinucleated cells formed in vitro from Paget's bone marrow express viral antigens. *Bone*. 1994;15:443–448.

Morrison AW. Genetic factors in otosclerosis. *Ann Royal Coll Surgeons*. 1967;41:2.

Morrison AW. Diseases of the otic capsule. In: Ballantyne J, Grove J, eds. *Scott Brown's Diseases of the Ear, Nose and Throat*. 4th ed. London: Butterworths; 1979:414.

Nager GT. Histopathology of otosclerosis. *Acta Otolaryngol*. 1969;89:341–362.

Nager GT. Osteogenesis imperfecta of the temporal bone and its relation to otosclerosis. *Ann Otol, Rhinol Laryngol*. 1988;97:585–593.

Nakamura S. Otosclerosis in Japan. *Acta Otolaryngol*. 1968;87:543–545.

Niedermeyer HP, Arnold W. Otosclerosis: A measles virus associated inflammatory disease. *Acta Otolaryngol*. 1995;115:300–303.

Nitze HR. Chromosome studies in otosclerosis. *Arch Klin Exp Ohren, Nasen, Kehlk–Heilk*. 1967;189:187.

Nizar R. The problem of otosclerosis in Indonesia. *Madj Kedokt Indonesia*. 1960; 10:398.

Nylen B. Histopathological investigations on the localization, number and activity and extent of otosclerotic foci. *J Laryngol Oto*. 1949;63:321–330.

Ogilvie R, Hall I. On the etiology of otosclerosis. *J Laryngol Otol*. 1962;76:841.

Petrovic A, Stutzmann J, Shambaugh GE. Experimental studies on pathology and therapy of otospongiosis. *Am J Otol*. 1985;6:43–50.

Rosen S, Bergman M, Plester D, El Mofty A, Satti MH. Presbyacusis study of a relatively noise free population in Sudan. *Ann Otolaryngol*. 1962;71:727–743.

Ruedi L. Pathogenesis of otosclerosis. *Acta Otolaryngol*. 1963;78:469.

Schiff M, Yoo TJ. Immunologic aspects of otologic disease: An overview. *Laryngoscope*. 1985;95:259–269.

Schmidt E. Erblichkeit und gravidatat bei der otosklerose. *Arch Ohren Nashen Kehlk–Heilk*. 1933;136:188.

Schneider–Schaulies J, Schneider–Schaulies S, ter Meulen V. Differential induction of cytokines by primary and persistent measles virus infections in human glial cells. *Virology*. 1993;195:219–228.

Schuknecht HF, Barber W. Histologic variants in otosclerosis. *Laryngoscope*. 1985;95: 1307–1317.

Schuknecht HF, Kirchner JC. Cochlear otosclerosis: Fact or fantasy. *Laryngoscope*. 1974;84:766–782.

Shambaugh GE. The diagnosis of otosclerosis. *Prog Otolaryngol*. 1952;1:395.

Shambaugh GE. Otosclerosis. *Proceedings of the International Congress of ORL*. Vol 1. Basel: Karger; 1961:367.

Shambaugh GE. *Surgery of the Ear*. 2nd ed. Philadelphia: WB Saunders; 1967:481.

Shea JJ, Farrior JB. Stapedectomy and round window closure. *Laryngoscope*. 1987;97:10–12.

Singhal SK, Mann SBS, Datta U, et al. Genetic correlation in otosclerosis. *Am J Otolaryngol*. 1999;20:102–105.

Sorenson MS, Nielson LP, Bretlau P, et al. The role of type II collagen autoimmunity in otosclerosis revisted. *Acta Otolaryngol*. 1988;105:242–247.

Takahara S, Sumida S, Fujimori H, Nagao N. A statistical survey of clinical otosclerosis encountered in Okayama University Medical School during 1955–1957. *J Otorhinolaryngol Soc Japan*. 1959;62:2271.

Tato JM, Tato JM Jr. Otosclerosis and races. *Ann Otol*. 1967;76:1018–1025.

Tato JM, Tato JM Jr. Quelques résultats des examens otologiques et audiologiques des indiens Sud Americans. *Acta Otolaryngol (Stockholm)*. 1969;67:277–280.

Thalmann I, Thallinger G, Thalmann R. Otosclerosis: A localized manifestation of a generalized connective tissue disorder? *Am J Otolaryngol*. 1987;8:308–316.

Thiers FA, Valvassori GE, Nadol JB. Otosclerosis of the cochlear capsule: Correlation of computerized tomography and histopathology. *Am J Otol*. 1999;20:93–95.

Tomek M, Brown MR, Mani SR, et al. Localization of a gene for otosclerosis to chromosome 15q–q26. *Human Molecular Genetics*. 1998;7:285–290.

Toynbee J. Otosclerosis. *Medico Surgical Transactions*. 1861;24:190.

Valvassori GE. Imaging of otosclerosis. *Otolaryngol Clin N Am*. 1993;26:359–371.

Walsh T. The effect of pregnancy on the deafness of otosclerosis. *Trans Am Acad Ophthalmol Otolaryngol*. 1954;58:420–425.

Walsh T. Influence of pregnancy on deafness. *Arch Otolaryngol*. 1954;69:334–336.

Wang PA, Merchant SN, McKenna MJ, Glynn RJ, Nadol JB. Does otosclerosis occur only in the temporal bone? *Am J Otol*. 1999;20:162–165.

Wayoff M, Chobaut JC, Raffoux JE, et al. Systeme HLA et otospongiose. *J Française Otorhinolaryngol*. 1979;28:299–301.

Weber MJ. The blue mantles in otosclerosis: A contribution to the pathology of the labyrinthine capsule. *Ann Otol, Rhinol Laryngol*. 1933;42:438–454.

Wiet ERJ. Patterns of ear disease in the southwestern American Indian. *Arch Otolaryngol*. 1979;105:381–385.

Witmaack K. Uber die sogennanteexperimentelle Huhnerotosklrose. *Acta Otolaryngol*. 1930;14:228.

Wolff AN. Otosclerosis: Hypothesis of its origin and progress. *Arch Otolaryngol (Chicago)*. 1950;58:853.

Yoo TJ, Stuart JM, Kang AH, et al. Type II collagen immunity in otosclerosis and Meniere's disease. *Science*. 1982;217:1153–1155.

Yoo TJ, Tomoda K, Stuart JM, Kang AH, Townes AS. Type II collagen induced autoimmune otospongiosis: A preliminary report. *Ann Otol, Rhinol Laryngol*. 1983;92:103–108.

Ziyeh S, Berlis A, Ross UH, et al. MRI of active otosclerosis. *Neuroradiology*. 1997;39:453–457.

*Chapter* *3*

# Physical Examination and Clinical Evaluation of the Patient with Otosclerosis

The patient with otosclerosis usually suffers from a gradually progressive hearing loss. This is usually bilateral and may be asymmetrical. Age of presentation is usually in the third or fourth decade. The patient will most likely be female, and if the patient has a family history of conductive deafness, the diagnosis of otosclerosis will be more likely. Patients will likely be soft spoken because they hear their own voice as louder as a result of bone conduction (Emmett 1993). Similarly, patients will complain of worsening hearing disability while eating. For female patients, the hearing disability often worsens with the onset of pregnancy.

A history for previous ear surgery should be elicited.

## PHYSICAL EXAMINATION

The entire auditory system should be evaluated thoroughly. The pinna and external auditory canals should be inspected, and any debris that might obscure the tympanic membrane should be carefully removed.

The tympanic membrane should be examined, preferably with the aid of the operating microscope. In particular, the tympanic membrane should be evaluated to rule out the presence of other disorders that could cause a conductive hearing loss. The presence of tympanosclerotic plaques on the tympanic membrane or thinning of the tympanic membrane could well point to tympanosclerosis as a cause of the conductive hearing loss, by causing fixation of the ossicular chain.

Fluid in the middle ear and barotrauma should be ruled out when eliciting a history as well as when conducting a physical exam. Chronic adhesive otitis media and tympanic membrane perforation, as well as cholesteatoma, if present, will be evident to the experienced otolaryngologist upon examination of the tympanic membrane under the microscope. On occasion a reddish blush will be evident. This is known as Schwartze's sign. This reddish blush is due to abnormal vascular shunts between the otosclerotic focus and the vessels on the promontory. This is a sign of an active otosclerotic focus and could be a contraindication for surgery.

## Use of the Pneumatic Otoscope

The pneumatic otoscope can help differentiate between malleus fixation and otosclerosis (Moon and Hahn 1978). If the malleus is fixed, the excursion of the tympanic membrane will be minimal when the bulb of the pneumatic otoscope is compressed. In otosclerosis, however, the excursion of the tympanic membrane may appear to be normal. This tool, though a subjective one, can in experienced hands identify the presence of malleus fixation.

## Tuning Fork Tests

Although audiological tests are now freely available and the degree of hearing loss can be evaluated, it is still necessary for the otolaryngologist to perform tuning fork tests in order to arrive at a reasonable idea as to the nature of the hearing loss and its severity. It is also a quick and, again in experienced hands, reliable way of assessing the type and nature of the hearing loss and can help compare the findings of the tuning fork with those found on pure tone and impedance audiometry. It should be remembered that pure tone and speech audiometry are subjective tests that can vary from one audiological laboratory to another.

The tuning forks used are 256, 512, and 1024 Hz. The tuning fork tests should be performed with all three tuning forks by both the audiologist and the otolaryngologist.

Rinne's test is a reliable method for ascertaining if the hearing loss is a conductive one. The tines of the tuning fork are placed 2 cm away from the external auditory canal, and the patient is asked to indicate when the sound of the vibrating tuning fork is no longer heard. This is evaluating air conduction of sound. When the patient indicates that he or she can no longer hear the tuning fork, the still vibrating fork is placed on the skin overlying the antral area of the mastoid. This evaluates bone conduction of sound. The patient is then asked if he or she can hear the sound of the vibrating tuning fork.

A Rinne's test is positive if air conduction is greater (longer) than bone conduction. It is negative if bone conduction is greater than air conduction. A negative Rinne's test indicates the presence of a conductive hearing loss. For a Rinne's test to be negative with a 512 Hz tuning fork, an air-bone gap of at least 30 to 45 dB is needed.

Weber's test is also useful in identifying the ear with the greater conductive hearing loss. When the tuning fork is placed on the middle of the forehead, the patient perceives the sound as louder in the ear with the greater conductive hearing loss. When a unilateral conductive hearing loss is present and the other ear is normal, the sound of the tuning fork will be heard (lateralizes) in the ear that has a conductive hearing loss. In situations of unilateral sensorineural hearing loss, the sound of the tuning fork is more audible in the normal ear than in the ear that has a sensorineural hearing loss.

### False-Negative Rinne's Test

A false-negative Rinne's test is obtained when a unilateral profound sensorineural hearing loss exists. Failure to recognize such a situation may lead the examiner to conclude that a conductive hearing loss exists. Masking the nontest (contralateral) ear with a Bárány noise box helps identify if a profound sensorineural hearing loss is present. Masking the nontest ear may fail to identify the sensorineural hearing loss in the tested ear if a conductive hearing loss is present in the nontest ear. Thus, the Rinne's test must be interpreted guardedly. In addition, a Rinne's test should be conducted in a soundproof room for correct interpretation. Rinne's and Weber's tests should be interpreted in conjunction with each other to arrive at an accurate conclusion.

## Absolute Bone Conduction (ABC) Test

An absolute bone conduction (ABC) test compares the patient's bone conduction with that of the examiner. The examiner in turn must have had his or her hearing thresholds previously examined by pure tone audiometry, and they should be normal.

In the test, the external auditory canal of the ear being tested is occluded. The tuning fork (512 Hz) is then placed over the patient's mastoid. The patient is asked to indicate when he or she can no longer hear the mastoid. The tuning fork is then transferred to the examiner's mastoid. If the patient can no longer hear the sound while the examiner can still hear the tuning fork, then the patient's absolute bone conduction is reduced. This usually indicates a sensorineural hearing loss.

In pure stapedial otosclerosis, the Rinne's test is negative. In unilateral or asymmetrical deafness, the Weber's test is lateralized to the more affected side, and the ABC test is normal. In pure cochlear otosclerosis, the Rinne's test is positive and the ABC test is reduced, the Weber's being lateralized to the better hearing ear. In combined otosclerosis, the Rinne's test is negative, and the ABC test is reduced.

## VESTIBULAR SYMPTOMS AND OTOSCLEROSIS

An association between vertigo and otosclerosis is well recognized. Clinical evidence has shown that otosclerotic patients have a vestibular involvement varying between 27 and 30% (Hulk and Jongkees 1950; Morales-Garcia 1972; Rasmussen 1949). Morales-Garcia (1972) reported that patients with sensorineural hearing loss had a greater vestibular involvement. He pointed out that cochlear involvement is not necessarily accompanied by vestibular compromise and that vestibular compromise can occur in the absence of cochlear involvement. Meniere's disease has been diagnosed in patients suffering from otosclerosis.

One common presentation that occurs is a true benign paroxysmal positional vertigo while the patient is lying on one side or while he or she is tilting the head to one side. Such patients were usually found to have large notches or loss of bone conduction over 2000 Hz. Transient episodes of vertigo, often positional, occur in patients with pure cochlear otosclerosis.

Two mechanisms have been postulated in the literature by which an otosclerotic focus could cause vertigo: (1) The otosclerotic focus could produce end organ or neural degeneration or both (Gussen 1973; Sando et al 1974). (2) Vertigo is produced when the otosclerotic focus comes in contact with the perilymph, which then results in a change in the biochemistry of the perilymph (Ghorayeb and Linthicum 1978).

There is a relationship between otosclerosis and endolymphatic hydrops (Johnsson et al 1982; Liston et al 1984). The exact mechanism is not clearly understood, although it does exist.

For patients suffering from Meniere's disease, McCabe (1966) recommended control of symptoms for at least 6 months before actively considering stapedectomy. This is because a markedly dilated saccule would lie very close to the stapedial footplate, thus serving as a contraindication for stapedectomy.

In their review of 228 patients of proven otosclerosis, Emmet and Shea (1989) found that one third had vertigo preoperatively. They concluded that patients had vestibular symptoms but did not suffer from endolymphatic hydrops could still undergo stapedectomy. Furthermore, not only can a successful stapedectomy be performed, but such patients experience relief from the vestibular symptoms following stapedectomy.

## TINNITUS

Tinnitus is also known to be associated with otosclerosis. The exact mechanism by which this occurs, however, is unclear at this time. The reported incidence was 70% (Wiet et al 1991). Tinnitus is common in those patients with severe sensorineural hearing loss combined with stapedial fixation. Tinnitus is frequently encountered in the older age group with combined otosclerosis and in those with an early age of onset and cochlear involvement. Tinnitus is not a contraindication for stapedectomy, and low-tone tinnitus may disappear after a well-performed stapedectomy. Sodium fluoride therapy may be helpful to gradually lessen the intensity of the tinnitus.

## SENSORINEURAL HEARING LOSS

The mechanism by which otosclerosis causes sensorineural hearing loss is not clearly established. The hypotheses responsible for this phenomenon are postulated as follows:

1. Liberation of toxic metabolites into the fluids of the inner ear (Causse and Chevance 1978; Nager 1969)

2. Vascular compromise and hypoxemia of the structures of the inner ear (Ruedi and Spondlin 1966)

3. Alteration of the mechanism of motion within the cochlear duct because of endosteal involvement of the cochlea (Linthicum et al 1975).

Lindsay and Beal (1966) found sensorineural hearing loss only in temporal bones with extensive, multifocal, active otosclerosis. Linthicum (1967) demonstrated a relationship between the degree of cochlear endosteal involvement, hyalinization of the spiral ligament, and sensorineural hearing loss. Balle and Linthicum (1984) reported the presence of sensorineural hearing loss in selected cases of otosclerosis without stapedial footplate fixation.

Cochlear otosclerosis is discussed in Chapter 6.

## DIFFERENTIAL DIAGNOSIS

### Tympanosclerosis

A patient with tympanosclerosis usually presents with a unilateral conductive hearing loss. The patient will give a history of multiple attacks of otitis media and may give a history of chronic otorrhea. If the tympanic membrane in such a patient has healed, the tympanic membrane will appear scarred or thinned out, or tympanosclerotic plaques will be seen on the tympanic membrane. On occasion the patient may give a history of previous ear surgery that failed to improve hearing. If a postaural scar is seen, this usually points to surgery for closure of a perforation. In such a patient tympanosclerosis would likely be present. This can only be confirmed by a tympanotomy, with careful inspection of the middle ear and careful evaluation of the mobility of the ossicles. Tympanosclerotic plaques will be seen crowding the ossicles, impairing their mobility. Nonetheless, tympanosclerosis is a clinical diagnosis that is made during a middle ear exploration even though a high index of suspicion may exist prior to surgery.

### Paget's Disease

Paget's disease may often be monostotic and may be confined only to the temporal bone. It is typically seen in the older patient and is associated with a sensorineural or mixed hearing loss. Sometimes vestibular symptoms are present. Paget's disease can often cause fixation of the stapes. More often it crowds the ossicles in the epitympanum. Cochlear involvement is found as the disease advances, and other bones of the body are also affected. Elevation of the serum alkaline phosphatase levels and involvement of other bones are typical of Paget's disease. The results of stapedectomy for Paget's disease are not as good as those for otosclerosis.

### Osteogenesis Imperfecta

Also known as van der Hoeve's syndrome, osteogenesis imperfecta is an autosomal dominant disorder with variable expression. The underlying disorder is one of faulty collagen maturation and poor bone formation. It presents as a triad of brittle bones, blue sclera, and hearing loss. Not all patients present with the triad of symptoms, with the hearing loss being a variable manifestation. Osteogenesis imperfecta results in a conductive hearing loss caused by stapedial footplate fixation.

### Ossicular Discontinuity

Ossicular discontinuity usually occurs following a head injury. In such a situation, the index of suspicion would be high, especially if the patient's hearing was normal prior to the head injury. If the patient also complains of dizziness, then subluxation of the footplate must be suspected; this should be treated as an emergency. Surgical repair is needed in such a circumstance.

### Osteopetrosis (Albers-Schönberg Disease)

This disease process causes a conductive hearing loss by bony overgrowth in the middle ear space and by congenital fixation of the ossicles in the attic. The other manifestations of this disease are much more serious and are fatal.

## Congenital Stapes Fixation

Bilateral congenital stapes fixation is a rare disorder. It is a sex-linked disease that manifests as bilateral mixed hearing loss. These patients also present with vestibular abnormalities such as absent or abnormal caloric responses. Family history is strongly positive in males (Jahn and Vernick 1986). Patients with congenital fixed footplates are associated with perilymph gushers at the time of stapedectomy. Such patients may therefore not be ideal candidates for stapedectomy. Strong family history, bilateral disease, and a history of perilymph gushers in other family members who may have undergone surgery upon the footplate point toward a congenitally fixed footplate.

## REFERENCES

Balle V, Linthicum FH. Histologically proven cochlear otosclerosis with pure sensorineural hearing loss. *Ann Otol, Rhinol Laryngol.* 1984;93:1–5.

Causse JR, Chevance LG. Sensorineural hearing loss due to cochlear otospongiosis: etiology. *Otolaryngol Clin N Am.* 1978;11:125–134.

Emmett JR. Physical examination and clinical evaluation of the patient with otosclerosis. *Otolaryngol Clin N Am.* 1993;26:353–357.

Emmett JR, Shea JJ. Vestibular dysfunction associated with otosclerosis. *Trans Am Otol Soc.* 1989;8:104–107.

Ghorayeb BY, Linthicum FH. Otosclerotic inner ear syndrome. *Ann Otol, Rhinol Laryngol.* 1978;87:85–90.

Gussen R. Otosclerosis and vestibular degeneration. *Arch Otolaryngol.* 1973;97: 484–487.

Hulk J, Jongkees LBW. Vestibular examination in cases of otosclerosis. *J Laryngol Otol.* 1950;64:126–130.

Jahn AF, Vernick D. Differential diagnosis. In: *Otosclerosis: Diagnosis and Treatment.* Alexandria, Va.: SIPAC American Academy of Otolaryngology—Head and Neck Surgery; 1986:10–15.

Johnsson LG, Hawkins JE, Rouse RC. Cochlear and otoconial abnormalities in capsular otosclerosis with hydrops. *Ann Otol, Rhinol, Laryngol.* 1982;91(suppl): 3–15.

Lindsay JR, Beal DD. Sensorineural deafness in otosclerosis: Observations on histopathology. *Ann Otol, Rhinol Laryngol.* 1966;75:436–457.

Linthicum FH. Pathology and pathogenesis of sensorineural deafness in otosclerosis. *ENT Digest.* 1967;29:51–56.

Linthicum FH, Filipo R, Brody S. Sensorineural hearing loss due to cochlear otospongiosis: Theoretical considerations of etiology. *Ann Otol, Rhinol Laryngol.* 1975; 84:544–551.

Liston SL, Paparella MM, Mancini F, Anderson JH. Otosclerosis and endolymphatic hydrops. *Laryngoscope.* 1984;94:1003–1007.

McCabe BF. Otosclerosis and vertigo. *Trans Pacific Coast Otol-Ophthalmol Soc.* 1966; 47:37–42.

Moon CN, Hahn M. Pneumatic otoscopy and impedance studies in middle ear diagnosis. *Laryngoscope.* 1978;88:1439–1448.

Morales-Garcia C. Cochleovestibular involvement in otosclerosis. *Acta Otolaryngol.* 1972;73:484–492.

Nager GT. Histopathology of otosclerosis. *Acta Otolaryngol.* 1969;89:341–362.

Rasmussen H. Vestibular function prior to and following operation for otosclerosis. *Arch Otolaryngol.* 1949;49:402–413.

Ruedi L, Spondlin H. Die Histologie der otosklerotischer Stapesankylose im Hinblick auf die chirurgischer Mobilization des Steibugels. *Z Ohrenheilk.* 1957;41:184.

Sando I, Hemenway WG, Miller DR, et al. Vestibular pathology in otosclerosis: Temporal bone histopathological report. *Laryngoscope.* 1974;84:593–605.

Wiet RJ, Causse JB, Shambaugh GE, Causse JR. Otosclerosis (otospongiosis). Alexandria, Va.: CME American Academy of Otolaryngology—Head and Neck Surgery; 1991:56–66.

# Chapter 4

# Audiological Evaluation of the Patient with Otosclerosis

The audiological pattern in otosclerosis is unique. The patterns of abnormalities can be directly explained by alterations in the middle ear transfer function produced by stapes fixation (Harrell 2002).

## PURE TONE AUDIOMETRY

Pure tone audiometry is the most basic test that should be performed with any patient presenting with impairment in hearing. It should be remembered, however, that it is a subjective test, and the results can vary from laboratory to laboratory. Nonetheless, it is the most important audiological test.

## AIR CONDUCTION

The most prominent audiological characteristics of otosclerosis are elicited with the use of low-frequency stimuli (Hannley 1993). The primary acoustic consequence of otosclerosis in its early stages is the increase in the stiffness reactance component of the total middle ear impedance. This results in a reduction of transmission effectiveness for low frequencies, as seen in elevated thresholds. Another effect is that the resonant frequency of the middle ear is elevated (Beales 1981).

In the early stages, a gradually progressive low-frequency conductive hearing loss is first seen. Initially, patients may be unaware of such a hearing impairment until it crosses the 25 dB range. The hearing loss may be confined to frequencies below 1000 Hz; high frequencies are typically unaffected at this stage. This characteristic rising audiogram configuration has been referred to as the "stiffness tilt."

As the footplate becomes completely fixed and the otosclerotic focus proliferates, a mass effect is added to the audiogram. The low-frequency hearing loss does not increase and appears to stabilize. The hearing loss progresses in the high frequencies, however, and there is a gradual widening of the air-bone gap. The audiogram configuration now changes to a flat pattern from the upward-sloping pattern that it had in the early stages. In the absence of cochlear involvement, the pure conductive hearing loss produced

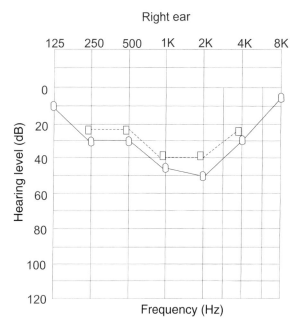

**Figure 4–1** Pure tone audiogram of a patient suffering from cochlear otosclerosis. The multiple sloping pattern gives it the appearance of a cookie bite. Dotted line = bone conduction. Solid line = air conduction.

by the complete stapes fixation is limited to 60 to 65 dB, with a maximum air-bone gap across the frequency range.

In cochlear otosclerosis, air conduction thresholds continue to worsen, and the loss starts to become mixed or sensorineural, with the high frequencies becoming severely affected. The typical pattern of cochlear otosclerosis in the early stages is the "cookie bite" pattern (Fig. 4–1), where the greatest degree of hearing loss occurs in the midfrequency hearing range and is characteristically a mixed hearing loss (Hannley 1993).

Tinnitus is usually present in a large percentage of patients. If the tinnitus is severe, it may interfere with the patient's ability to respond reliably to pure tone testing. Usage of pulsed or warbled tones may help the patient to identify tinnitus from pure tone test stimuli when being tested.

## BONE CONDUCTION

Although air conduction curves give an indication of the hearing thresholds, and its configuration may give valuable clues to the diagnosis of otosclerosis in its early stages, bone conduction audiometry is of great value in the diagnosis of otosclerosis and in the selection of patients for surgery. Bone conduction is especially useful when testing patients suffering from otosclerosis. It reveals characteristics that are typical of otosclerosis, and it also helps to reveal the amount of cochlear reserve in each ear. This helps to determine if stapedial or cochlear otosclerosis is present. This in turn helps the surgeon make a decision as to which ear he or she should operate and helps predict optimum postoperative results.

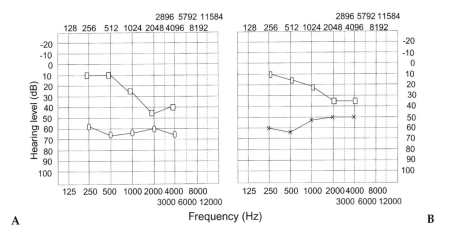

Frequency (Hz)

A                                                                                   B

**Figure 4–2** **(A)** Pure tone audiogram of a patient suffering from fenestral otosclerosis. Note Carhart's notch at 2000 Hz. **(B)** Pure tone audiogram of a patient who has a central perforation. There is no notch at 2000 Hz. *(Adapted from Beales, PH. Otosclerosis. Bristol; John Wright and Sons: 1981. Used with permission.)*

Carhart's notch (Fig. 4–2) is thought to be typical of otosclerosis (Carhart 1950, 1962). It is characterized by the elevation of bone conduction thresholds of approximately 5 dB at 500 Hz, 10 dB at 1000 Hz, 15 dB at 2000 Hz, and 5 dB at 4000 Hz. It was previously thought that this was due to the inertial component of bone conduction caused by stapes fixation. The contribution of the inertial component is maximal for frequencies below 800 Hz, however; thus, a greater loss for bone-conducted low frequencies might be predicted. Yet this is not borne out by clinical observation. Another more plausible explanation is that fixation of the stapes disrupts normal ossicular resonance, which in humans is around 2000 Hz. Furthermore, the normal compression mode of bone conduction is disturbed because of the relative perilymph immobility caused by stapes fixation (Tonndorf 1972). Carhart's notch is a mechanical artifact and is not a true representation of cochlear reserve. Evidence that it is an artifact is seen in overclosure following stapes surgery.

Cross-checks on the validity of bone conduction thresholds include careful consideration of the masking levels. The sensorineural acuity level (SAL) test is used to resolve masking dilemmas.

It must be appreciated that Carhart's notch occurs in any condition that reduces the inertial vibration of the stapes footplate during bone conduction stimulation. One such condition is otosclerosis. It would be incorrect, however, to assume that this is the only condition that can cause Carhart's notch (Fig. 4–3).

Carhart (1950) gave four postulates to indicate that stapes fixation induces mechanical modifications in the bone conduction audiogram:

1. In the Bing test in clinical otosclerosis, there is no shift in loudness when the meatus is occluded or when pressure is varied, as is seen in normal hearing and in sensorineural hearing loss. It is probable that the Bing test is negative in otosclerosis and on other forms of deafness because the

33

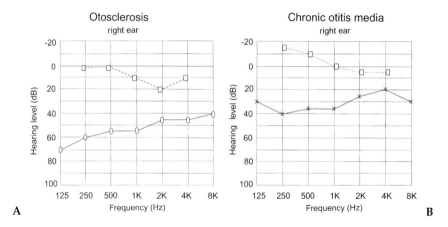

**Figure 4–3** Pure tone audiogram of two siblings who have a history of otosclerosis. Note the notch at 2000 Hz typical of otosclerosis. *(Adapted from Beales, PH. Otosclerosis. Bristol; John Wright and Sons: 1981. Used with permission.)*

middle ear element of bone conduction is attenuated by the middle ear element of hearing loss.

2. It is unusual to find a patient with otosclerosis whose bone conduction thresholds are normal.

3. Surgery improves bone conduction thresholds, and the Carhart's notch disappears following surgery.

4. Animal experiments producing stapes fixation cause bone conduction thresholds to become poorer.

It was thought that there was an abrupt shift in bone conduction thresholds, and that this may reach its full magnitude when stapes fixation has progressed to the stage at which it causes a mild air conduction loss. Beales (1981) disagreed, finding evidence of a slowly progressive increase in the size of the Carhart's notch. In chronic otitis media, Carhart's notch-like effects may occur, but they are much less prominent than those seen in otosclerosis.

Not all high-frequency bone conduction losses are artifacts. Cochlear otosclerosis is characterized by the presence of mixed or sensorineural hearing losses in which the air-bone gap is minimal. If the air conduction and bone conduction levels are roughly parallel, the elevated bone conduction thresholds probably represent a sensorineural hearing loss.

Keleman and Linthicum (1969) discovered that the severity and configuration of the pure tone audiogram do not match the frequency for those areas of the cochlea. Sensorineural hearing losses are most commonly associated with basal turn involvement and are invariably present with endosteal layer involvement. Sensorineural hearing loss varies directly with hyalinization of the spiral ligament.

## Clinical Value of Bone Conduction Audiometry

In otosclerosis, there is a characteristic bone conduction curve that helps the clinician distinguish otosclerosis from other causes of conductive hearing losses. The clinician can determine with accuracy the degrees of sensorineural reserve by correcting the bone conduction audiogram for mechanical distortion due to stapes fixation. Stated another way, it is possible to more precisely determine a patient's hearing loss due to secondary cochlear loss by making allowance for the Carhart's notch when interpreting bone conduction thresholds.

## FALSE LATERALIZATION

The false lateralization phenomenon occurs during a Weber's test when the sound is referred to the other ear. This error is common when bone conduction audiometry is performed without masking; under these circumstances, the bone threshold in the worst affected ear may seem to be better than it really is, by approximately 10 dB or more, as the patient is hearing the sound in the other ear.

## HYPERDISTRACTIBILITY

In some cases, the introduction of a masking noise creates serious interference with the response of the ear under test, even though the sound is not strong enough to produce cross-masking in this ear. Such patients do poorly even though the noise is too weak to be producing true masking in the test ear. This effect is termed *central masking*.

## SHADOW RESPONSE

In some patients with whom hearing losses are severe, efforts to mask the contralateral ear become ineffective. This situation arises because effective masking is reduced at each frequency by the amount of the air conduction loss in the masked ear at that frequency. To illustrate this point, a masking noise that causes a 50 dB threshold shift in a normal ear will produce only about 10 dB of shift in an ear with a hearing loss of 40 dB. This same noise will not cause any threshold shift in an ear where the air conduction loss exceeds 50 dB. This same noise will not cause any threshold shift in an ear where the air conduction loss exceeds 50 dB. There is also the possibility of cross-masking when the noise is increased even more in order to try to mask the ear, only to find that the masking noise has crossed the head and is now masking the test ear.

## MASKING

When conductive hearing losses are present, it is important that masking levels are appropriate and adequate. The goal of masking is to raise the threshold of the nontest ear so that the sensitivity of the test ear can be evaluated in isolation. Inadequate masking leads to participation of the nontest ear, resulting in incorrect levels of hearing estimates. Excessive masking levels lead to crossover of the masking to the test ear, leading to an underestimation of its cochlear reserve. Correct masking is difficult to achieve when moderate conductive losses exist. In these instances, the use of insert earphones for masking and the confirmation of thresholds by SAL may be necessary.

## SUMMARY OF PURE TONE AUDIOMETRY

In the early stages of otosclerosis, a low-frequency conductive hearing loss is found. As the severity of the disease progresses, the hearing loss increases in severity and changes in its configuration. Carhart's notch is a mechanical artifact of stapes fixation and is characteristic of otosclerosis. It disappears with successful closure of the air-bone gap. Bone conduction thresholds become progressively elevated in the high frequencies in cochlear otosclerosis. Adequate masking techniques are necessary when evaluating a patient with otosclerosis.

## IMPEDENCE AUDIOMETRY

Impedance audiometry has three components: tympanometry, static compliance, and acoustic reflexes.

### Tympanometry

The tympanogram is a graphic representation of the change in acceptance of sound energy through the middle ear as a function of air pressure applied to a hermetically sealed ear canal. Stated another way, tympanometry is the measurement of the tympanic membrane compliance in response to variations of air pressure in the external auditory canal. By varying the pressure in the external auditory canal, the point at which the tympanic membrane has maximum freedom to vibrate in response to a pure tone is when air pressure equals that in the middle ear.

Various schema have been proposed for classifying tympanograms. The classification proposed by Jerger (1970) (Fig. 4–4) is one of the more popular classifications and is used by the authors of this book. There are five types, described as types A, $A_s$, $A_d$, B, and C. The distinguishing feature of the entire A category (types A, $A_s$, $A_d$) is a clearly defined peak of the function, which occurs in the range of +100 daPa (atmospheric pressure). The tympanometric peak demonstrates the presence of air in the middle ear space. The location of the peak on the pressure axis serves as an indicator of middle ear air pressure relative to ambient air pressure; thus, it indirectly indicates the position of the tympanic membrane. The height of the tympanogram (the base–peak compliance difference) reflects the mobility of the middle ear apparatus, including the tympanic membrane, the ossicles, and the inherent stiffness of the air enclosed in the external ear canal and that of the air in the middle ear space.

Middle ear aeration is not affected in otosclerosis. The middle ear pressure is zero or atmospheric. A clear peak that remains within the normal range of 100 daPa, type A category, characterizes the tympanograms of patients suffering from otosclerosis. Further subdivision is decided on the basis of the base–peak compliance difference. This value will depend on several factors, one of which is the condition of the tympanic membrane. Thus, a stiffened tympanic membrane caused by tympanosclerosis will result in a stiff ($A_s$) tympanogram. A flaccid tympanic membrane would result in a deep ($A_d$) configuration.

In the case of stapedial otosclerosis, the height of the tympanometric peak decreases.

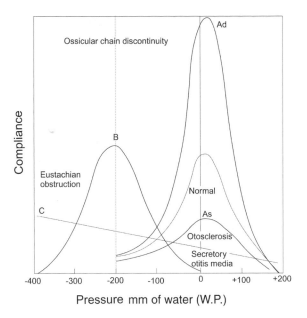

**Figure 4–4** Tympanograms according to the classification of Jerger. Ad = tympanogram associated with ossicular discontinuity. As = tympanogram associated with otosclerosis. (*Adapted from Beales, PH. Otosclerosis. Bristol; John Wright and Sons: 1981. Used with permission.*)

## Static Compliance

The static compliance is calculated by subtracting the compliance at +200 daPa from the total compliance when the pressure is equilibrated across the tympanic membrane, and energy transfer is at a peak:

$$\text{static compliance} = \text{peak compliance} - \text{compliance}_{200\text{daPa}}$$

Normal static compliance values fall in the range of 0.3 to 1.6 cc. Values lower than 0.3 cc are considered abnormally low, indicative of increased stiffness in the conductive mechanism. If the compliance is greater than 0.6 cm$^3$, it is probable that the footplate of the stapes will be relatively thin. If the compliance is less than 0.2 cm$^3$, then there is a possibility that the footplate will be fairly thick; the footplate may even be obliterative. If the hearing loss is symmetrical, this information may be helpful in selecting which ear should be operated upon.

## Acoustic Reflexes

The principle of acoustic reflexes is this: the middle ear muscles contract reflexively to a stimulus. The stiffness of the entire middle ear system is increased, resulting in a corresponding decrease in transmission efficiency for a low-frequency tone. The earliest evidence of otosclerosis is often the appearance of a diphasic pattern (Bel et al 1976). The diphasic reflex is characterized by brief increases in compliance that occur at the onset and at the termination of the stimulus when the probe is in the affected ear (Flottorp and Djupesland 1970).

Bel at al (1976) account for this phenomenon by postulating that, although the anterior footplate may be fixed to the oval window, the elasticity of the involved footplate and crura allows the posterior portion of the footplate to move independent of the anterior portion of the footplate, creating the onset compliance change. The elasticity of the footplate returns it to its resting position, where it remains until the pull of the tendon of the stapedius is relaxed, allowing another brief change in compliance at the offset of the signal.

As the stapes becomes progressively fixed, the ipsilateral and contralateral acoustic reflexes are affected, even though the stapes fixation may be unilateral. This causes the impedance matching function of the ear to be less effective; as a result of the inefficient impedance match, the signal is attenuated before it arrives at the cochlea for the first stage of the reflex arc.

In the early stages of the disease, acoustic reflex abnormalities may be apparent only when the probe is placed in the affected ear, which produces a "vertical pattern" in the convention created by Jerger and Jerger (1977). As the degree of hearing loss increases, contralateral reflexes become abnormal and produce the "inverted L pattern" in which only the ipsilateral reflex in the unaffected ear remains observable.

## NONACOUSTIC REFLEXES

Nonacoustic reflexes may be produced by tactile stimulation. This may help in distinguishing malleus and stapes fixation. The nonacoustic reflex is generally believed to be related to tensor tympani activity and is characterized by its appearance as part of a generalized startle reflex, by rapid habituation to repeated stimuli, and by changes in compliance opposite to those seen with stapedial contraction. The tactile stimulation may take the form of directing a jet of air to the ipsilateral cornea or by lightly stroking the tragus. If the acoustic reflex is absent or abnormal but the nonacoustic reflex is normal, the fixation site can be inferred to be at the stapes (Hannley 1993). If the acoustic and nonacoustic reflexes are absent or abnormal, however, then malleus fixation or generalized ossicular fixation may be suspected (Klockhoff and Anderson 1960). Normal tympanograms, static compliance accompanied by acoustic reflex abnormalities such as diphasic reflex, elevated thresholds, and absent reflexes in one or both ears are the typical pattern of otosclerosis in its early phases. As the stapes footplate gets more firmly fixed, the tympanogram becomes shallower, with a corresponding decrease in static compliance.

## SPEECH AUDIOMETRY

Speech audiometry (Fig. 4–5) completes the audiological battery of tests. Persons suffering from sensorineural hearing loss will complain that they are unable to comprehend speech in a noisy background. Those who suffer from a conductive hearing loss, however, will hear better in a noisy background. This is the paradox known as the paracusis of Willis. This occurs because most speakers raise the level of their voices in order to be heard by

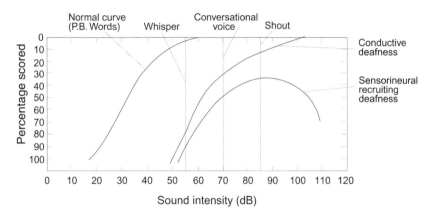

**Figure 4–5** Speech audiometry plotting. *(Adapted from Beales, PH. Otosclerosis. Bristol; John Wright and Sons: 1981.Used with permission.)*

themselves and their listeners (the Lombard effect), and in so doing cross the thresholds of those who have a conductive hearing loss. The listener's conductive hearing loss attenuates the background noise, leaving the speaker's voice more audible through an apparent improvement in the signal to noise ratio.

Spondee reception threshold, also known as the speech reception threshold (SRT), is the first test. In the presence of a conductive hearing loss, the SRT coincides with the three-frequency pure tone average (500 Hz, 1000 Hz, and 2000 Hz) within a range of 5 dB. The speech discrimination score (SDS) is a measure of word identification accuracy. SDS as measured by phonetically balanced words falls within the normal range of 90 to 100% at suprathreshold levels. Speech discrimination scores fall when there is a sensorineural component to the hearing loss. Thus, poor discrimination scores would indicate that the prognosis would be poor following surgery. Such patients would likely benefit more from hearing aid amplification.

## OTOACOUSTIC EMISSIONS

Otoacoustic emissions were first described by Kemp (1978). One study found that transient evoked otoacoustic emissions (TEOAEs) recorded from patients with otosclerosis have a very low amplitude and may not be observable above the recording noise floor in the presence of relatively minor amounts of conductive hearing loss. At this time, otoacoustic emissions have limited value in otosclerotic lesions with conductive hearing loss because of extreme vulnerability to middle ear transmission inefficiencies and a lack of specificity (Hannley 1993). Future research, however, may help in early identification of cochlear otosclerosis.

## VESTIBULAR TESTS

Vestibular tests become necessary in otosclerosis only when the patient also presents with vertigo. Causse and Causse (1991) described three types of vestibular dysfunction that are associated with otosclerosis. They postulated that vertigo occurs in these patients because of the release of toxic enzymes.

According to Causse and Causse, type 1 is characterized by mild dysequilibrium without a rotatory component. Caloric tests are normal. In type 2, attacks of acute rotational vertigo are experienced and may be accompanied by tinnitus and fluctuating sensorineural hearing loss. Paradoxically, the caloric tests may be normal in these patients. In the type 3 category, Meniere's disease and cochlear otosclerosis coexist.

## SUMMARY

Audiometry is a necessary tool to confirm and document the presence of otosclerosis. Otosclerosis presents in a unique and typical way. Pure stapedial otosclerosis has a unique signature, which can be recognized on pure tone and impedance audiometry. Accurate reliable audiometric tests that can be replicated help the clinician decide on the appropriate form of treatment for otosclerosis. Should surgery be agreed upon as the treatment, audiometric tests can help the surgeon decide which ear should be operated and help predict the outcome of such a surgery.

## REFERENCES

Beales PH. Functional evaluation of hearing. In: *Otosclerosis*. Bristol: John Wright and Sons; 1981:30–50.

Bel J, Causse JR, Michaux P, et al. Mechanical explanation of the on-off effect (diphasic impedance change) in otospongiosis. *Audiology*. 1976;15:128–130.

Carhart R. Clinical applications of bone conduction audiometry. *Arch Otolaryngol*. 1950;51:798–802.

Carhart R. Effects of stapes fixation on bone conduction responses. In: Schuknecht HF, ed. *International Symposium on Otosclerosis*. Boston: Little, Brown; 1962:175.

Causse JR, Causse JB. Clinical features and epidemiology of otospongiosis–otosclerosis. In: Wiet R, Causse JB, Shambaugh G, et al, eds. *Otosclerosis (Otospongiosis)*. Alexandria, Va.: American Academy of Otolaryngology—Head and Neck Surgery Foundation; 1991:56.

Flottorp G, Djupesland G. Diphasic impedance change and its applicability in clinical work. *Acta Otolaryngol*. 1970;263:200–205.

Hannley MT. Audiologic characteristics of the patient with otosclerosis. *Otolaryngol Clin N Am*. 1993;26:373–387.

Harrell RW. Pure tone evaluation. In: Katz J, ed. *Handbook of Clinical Audiology*. 5th ed. Philadelphia: Lippincott Williams and Wilkins; 2002:71–87.

Jerger J. Clinical experience with impedance audiometry. *Arch Otolaryngol*. 1970;92: 311–320.

Jerger J, Jerger S. Diagnostic value of crossed versus uncrossed acoustic reflexes: Eighth nerve and brain stem disorders. *Arch Otolaryngol*. 1977;103:445–448.

Keleman G, Linthicum F. Labyrinthine otosclerosis. *Acta Otolaryngol*. 1969;253(suppl): 1–68.

Kemp DT. Stimulated acoustic emissions from within the human auditory system. *J Acoustic Soc Am*. 1978;64:1386–1390.

Klockhoff I, Anderson H. Reflex activity in the tensor tympani muscle recorded in man. *Acta Otolaryngol*. 1960;51:184–187.

Tonndorf J. Bone conduction. In: Tobias J, ed. *Foundations of Modern Auditory Theory*. New York: Academic Press; 1972:175.

# Chapter *5*

# Radiological Imaging of Otosclerosis

Computed tomography (CT) scanning has replaced multidirectional to-mography in general and in the diagnosis of otosclerosis in particular. Be-cause most of the changes that occur are subtle, however, even CT scan-ning at this time may miss such findings. Magnetic resonance imaging (MRI) has had a limited role as yet in the imaging of otosclerosis. CT study should be performed with a modern apparatus using an extended gray scale up to 4000 Hounsfield units, small collimation, and a pixel size no more than 0.25 mm.

## FENESTRAL OTOSCLEROSIS

### Is CT Scanning Necessary?

Fenestral otosclerosis is a clinical diagnosis made on the basis of patient his-tory, family history, otoscopy, tuning fork tests, and audiometry. A CT scan can visualize the extent of the pathology of the oval window (Fig. 5–1); it is best used, however, in situations where patients present with mixed deaf-ness or with cochlear otosclerosis.

In active otosclerosis, the poorly calcified foci may not be recognizable. The margin of the oval window becomes decalcified, so that the oval win-dow seems larger than normal. In an inactive focus, the oval window may become narrowed, and in advanced cases it may be obliterated. Occasion-ally CT studies can be used to confirm a clinical diagnosis, and in those pa-tients with bilateral disease, CT scanning can help select the ear to be oper-ated upon.

### Postoperative Status

CT scanning is useful in evaluating patients postoperatively in situations where a hearing loss following an initial improvement has occurred. This is applicable to metallic prostheses (Fig. 5–2), because CT scans demonstrate if the prosthesis is in place or not. It should be remembered that because of volume averaging artifacts, the prosthesis may not be seen, or it may appear thicker than it actually is. Ultimately, the best way to check if the prosthesis is in place or not is by reexploring the middle ear.

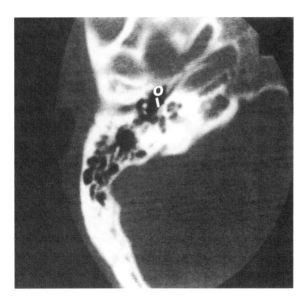

**Figure 5–1** High-resolution CT scan showing fenestral otoclerotic focus (O) anterior to the oval window. This was confirmed audiologically as well as surgically.

## COCHLEAR OTOSCLEROSIS

The normal otic capsule appears as a sharply defined homogeneously dense bony shell outlining the cochlea. Otosclerotic foci arise from the endochondral layer of the otic capsule and may be single or multiple. Large or multiple foci that merge with one another cause extensive demineralization. A typical sign of cochlear otosclerosis is the formation of a double ring effect

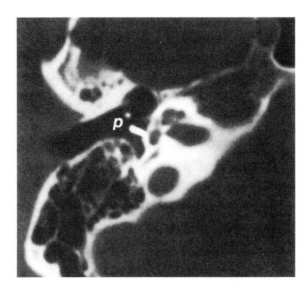

**Figure 5–2** CT scan in the postoperative period showing a metallic stapes prosthesis (p).

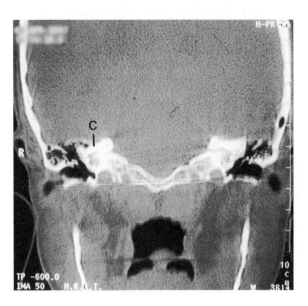

**Figure 5–3**  CT scan of the temporal bones in the coronal plane showing bilateral cochlear otosclerosis (C).

due to multiple interconnected foci within the otic capsule. Active foci appear as areas of demineralization, and inactive foci appear as areas of denser bone (Fig. 5–3). Therefore, CT scanning is useful in diagnosing cochlear otosclerosis only when the focus is in the active phase. In the sclerotic (inactive) phase, CT scanning may not be useful (Chole and McKenna 2001; Thiers et al 1999). Even large otosclerotic lesions may go undetected. CT scanning does have an important benefit: if a large patent cochlear aqueduct is present, a scan can alert the surgeon to the presence of a potential perilymph gusher (Swartz and Harnsberger 1992; Valvassori 1977). It can help alert the surgeon to the presence of other abnormalities or variations of normal anatomy such as a dehiscent jugular bulb.

CT scanning helps rule out other common causes of sensorineural hearing loss as well. When the otosclerotic focus involves the otic capsule, the density and outline of the cochlea are altered. At present, however, CT scanning is the only method to exclude or confirm the diagnostic suspicion of pure cochlear otosclerosis or far advanced otosclerosis. The reported (Mafee, Henrikson, et al 1985; Miura et al 1996; Swartz et al 1984) sensitivity of CT scan aiding a diagnosis of pure otosclerosis or far advanced otosclerosis ranges from 34 to 90%. More recent studies (Mafee, Valvassori, et al 1985), however, have claimed a higher percentage of detection of fenestral otosclerosis.

Valvasorri (1966, 1993) found that three factors must be considered when imaging cochlear otosclerosis on CT scanning. For the otosclerotic focus to be detected,

1. The focus must be greater than 1 mm in diameter; otherwise it will not be detected.

2. The density of the focus must differ from the rest of the otic capsule. That is why active (areas of demineralization) foci are easier to detect than inactive (sclerotic) foci.

3. The normal labyrinthine otic capsule is very dense. Sclerotic foci can be detected only when they are close to the periosteal or endosteal surfaces of the otic capsule.

The radiographic appearance of the otosclerotic lesion varies with the stage of maturation of the disease. Typical of cochlear otosclerosis is the formation of a double ring effect due to multiple foci merging with each other in the cochlea. When active and inactive foci appear together, a mosaic picture characterized by areas of decreased density with areas of increased density is seen. Finally, CT scanning must be correlated with clinical and audiological data to make a correct diagnosis. Further improvements in CT scanning, including better collimation and decreased pixel size, will produce images of higher definition.

## THE ROLE OF CT SCANNING IN FAMILIAL VERSUS SPORADIC OTOSCLEROSIS

In their retrospective study of 211 patients, Shin et al (2001) reported that in familial (hereditary) otosclerosis, radiologic signs are always present and may precede clinical expression of the disease. It was less sensitive, however, for those who were suffering from otosclerosis without any family history (sporadic otosclerosis) of otosclerosis. A family history of otosclerosis was found in 24.2% of their patients. The radiologic findings differed between patients with a sporadic form of the disease and patients who had a familial form of the disease. In the familial form, the lesions were more often detectable, bilateral, and severe. Their findings led to the assumption that fenestral otosclerosis occurs more in the sporadic form, whereas more extensive lesions on CT scanning seem to indicate the familial forms.

The real value of CT scanning lies in the treatment of far advanced otosclerosis when cochlear implantation is being actively considered. If the cochlear lumen is not clearly seen because of new bone formation, such patients are thought to be unsuitable candidates for cochlear implantation (Ruckenstein et al 2001).

In a study published by Shin et al (2001) of a survey of 437 cases (386 patients), the relationship between bone thresholds and extension of the otosclerotic foci within the otic capsule was studied by means of CT scanning. The patients were divided into two groups: those who had fenestral otosclerosis (group A) and those who had a pericochlear focus (group B). Data from both groups were then compared with those of a control group (group C) for whom CT scans showed no focus in the cochlea. A pericochlear focus was reported in 53 examinations. Their findings revealed that bone conduction thresholds were lower in group A than in the control group, but the difference was not significant. Bone thresholds were lower in group B than in the controls, and the difference was significant. The authors concluded that lower bone thresholds were associated with extension of the otosclerotic focus within the otic capsule.

## CT DENSITOMETRY

Quantitative data of the involvement of the cochlear capsule is plotted by using CT densitometry, as described by Valvasorri (1993). The cochlea is identified in the scout digitalized image, and six to eight axial sections at 1 mm increments are taken. Densitometry data are then collected from two CT scan sections taken at different levels.

Densitometric data are collected from two axial CT scans. The lower section passes through the basal turn of the cochlea and the round window niche (sites at which otosclerotic foci commonly occur). The upper section crosses the modiolus, exposing all three coils of the cochlea. Readings in Hounsfield units are taken as the cursor moves along the various areas of the cochlea just described. Readings are taken in normal patients with normal hearing and then compared with those in whom otosclerosis, especially cochlear otosclerosis, is suspected. Variations of density exceeding standard deviations of 10 to 15% for each point indicate cochlear involvement (Valvassori 1993). Thus, CT densitometry studies depend on comparisons between normal patients and those suffering from otosclerosis.

CT densitometry is thus an objective approach to the identification of otosclerotic foci in the cochlear capsule. It helps determine if the disease is active or inactive. Densitometry also helps in the evaluation of the disease, especially following fluoride therapy. Densitometric curves similar to those of otosclerosis occur in Paget's disease, osteogenesis imperfecta, and tertiary syphilis.

## THE ROLE OF MRI IN OTOSCLEROSIS

Valvassori (1993) has reported a new MR protocol for patients who have a positive Schwartze's sign. He observed a faint blush (enhancement) within the demineralized areas of the capsule. Although MRI has the potential to be used for examination of the lumen of the cochlea, especially for those patients who are preparing to undergo cochlear implantation (Berrettini et al 2002), at this time its use in fenestral and cochlear otosclerosis is limited.

MRI with gadolinium seems to be able to detect active otosclerotic foci in the labyrinthine capsule (Berrettini et al 2002). These appear as contrast enhanced areas in T1-weighted images with gadolinium. These authors acknowledge that it is difficult to differentiate the enhancement caused by the active otosclerotic focus from the normal enhancement resulting from the tympanic segment of the facial nerve (possible false-positive outcomes) (Sakai et al 2000). Furthermore, MRI cannot quantify the activity of the disease.

MRI is contraindicated in the postoperative stage for fear of dislodgment of the prosthesis, especially if the prosthesis is metallic. There is the possibility of vibration, dislodgment, or heating of the prosthesis with the accompanying possibility of sensorineural hearing loss (Syms and Petermann 2000).

Superimposition CT scanning and MRI (Ross et al 1995) may provide improvements in detection.

## SINGLE PHOTON EMISSION COMPUTED TOMOGRAPHY (SPECT) IN OTOSCLEROSIS

In CT scanning, the density of the otosclerotic focus is variable, and the active otosclerotic focus can be visualized only when the density loss is more than 200 Hounsfield units, whereas the inactive or sclerotic focus, being isodense with the normal osseous tissue, is detectable when the apposition of new otosclerotic focus causes irregularity or thickening of the otic capsule (Guneri et al 1996; Huizing and de Groot 1987; Shin et al 2000;). In tympanocochlear scintigraphy (TCS), the bone turnover caused by the otosclerotic focus can be detected using a radiopharmaceutical agent such as Tc 99m diphosphonate, which undergoes higher adsorption on immature (hydrated) than on mature (crystalline) hydroxyapatite (Bornemann et al 1981; Bornemann et al 1982; Ross et al 1993, 1995; Ziheh et al 1997). A major limitation of TCS is the absence of clear anatomic landmarks so that the distribution of the radioactive agent can be precisely located. SPECT scintigraphy is a dynamic technique that allows the study of bone metabolic activity by detecting the distribution of diphosphonate in petrous bone while also providing quantification of the radioactivity (Berrettini et al 2002). In addition to providing a semiquantitative analysis of metabolic activity as in tomographic techniques, it improves image contrast because it focuses on a thin slice of the structure and thus provides better location of anatomic landmarks. This allows the distribution of the radioactive agent to be located precisely.

To improve the ability of TCS to detect and localize otosclerotic foci, a correlation study must be performed between metabolic patterns and conventional radiographs or high-resolution CT scans (Ross et al 1996). To date, experimental and clinical studies of TCS have examined some temporal bones and only restricted and often undefined groups of otosclerotic patients without control groups.

A study was conducted by Berrettini and colleagues (2002) on the sensitivity of SPECT in 36 patients with surgically confirmed otosclerosis using controls. A cutoff value of 1.35 scintigraphic uptake index (UI) was used, and only 2 out of 72 ears in the otosclerotic group gave a false-negative outcome. Although the otosclerotic disease was bilateral in both patients, the UI was above the cutoff value in only one ear of each patient. Only 1 of 24 ears in the control group gave a false-positive result. The authors therefore concluded that SPECT appears to be very sensitive in differentiating otosclerotic bone from normal bone.

It was noted that the UI values of the otosclerotic patients had a varied range. This was attributed to the different stages of the disease; lower values were associated with low bone turnover, indicating inactive disease, and higher values were associated with high bone turnover associated with active disease. The mean UI value was 2.214 in otosclerotic patients, whereas in the control group it was 1.131. This difference was found to be statistically significant.

In bilateral disease, no statistical difference was found between the UI values for both ears of the same subject. Berrettini et al (2002) found that this confirmed that otosclerosis is indeed a bilateral disease. It was interesting to note that in this study the authors found three patients with clinical impairment also had high UI values on the side with normal hearing. They concluded that such findings could be explained by the fact that SPECT allows the detection of pathologic increases of bone metabolism even in the absence of clinical manifestations of the underlying process.

When the UI values were considered in relation to gender, no significant differences could be found. When age and gender findings were correlated, however, the authors noted that women under 45 years of age had a mean UI value that was higher than that of men in the same age group, whereas for women and men older than 45, the values were almost the same. They found this to be in keeping with the observations found on histopathology. The uptake of the bony labyrinth in relation to age revealed a higher uptake in younger patients. Again, these findings were consistent with those of literature where active foci are more likely to be associated in younger patients (Nager 1969).

Comparison of SPECT alterations with the severity of sensorineural hearing loss in younger versus older patients revealed a statistically significant correlation in the younger patients. This was found to indicate an increase in bone turnover, increased metabolic activity, and increased incidence of sensorineural hearing loss.

Berrettini et al (2002) thus concluded that SPECT presented a valid imaging technique that detected and localized otosclerotic foci. SPECT helped to quantify the disease and was also a cost-effective method. The primary disadvantage of SPECT was the length of the examination. This was because an interval of 3 hours is required between the injection of the isotope and the acquisition of data on the accumulation of radioisotope in the bone. SPECT was found to have a sensitivity of 97.2%. At this time, it is the only method that provides structural as well as functional data of the labyrinth of otosclerotic patients.

## SUMMARY

CT scanning has limited value in the diagnosis of fenestral otosclerosis because fenestral otosclerosis remains largely a clinical diagnosis. CT scanning does have potential in the diagnosis of cochlear otosclerosis. It can help in evaluating the response of the patient to fluoride therapy. CT scanning is more sensitive in active disease, especially if the patient is suffering from an inherited type of otosclerosis. CT densitometry has useful applications and needs to be developed further. CT scanning, though having limited value in fenestral otosclerosis, has one large benefit: if a large patent cochlear aqueduct is present, it helps alert the surgeon for a potential perilymph gusher. CT scanning is mandatory in far advanced otosclerosis, especially if cochlear implantation is being considered.

MRI is of limited value at this time. In the postoperative period, MRI is contraindicated because, if the prosthesis is metallic, it runs the risk of being dislodged or heated or undergoing catastrophic vibration, with the accompanying risk of sensorineural hearing loss.

Single photon emission CT scanning (SPECT) is a recent advance. It provides structural and functional information of the labyrinth in those patients suffering from otosclerosis. It was also found useful in quantifying the disease by being able to differentiate otosclerosis from normal bone and from active and inactive foci.

In conclusion, it may be said that most estimates of sensitivity imaging techniques for otosclerosis are based on correlations with diagnostic data obtained only on clinical grounds.

## REFERENCES

Berrettini S, Ravecca F, Volterrani D, et al. Single photon emission computed tomography in otosclerosis: Diagnostic accuracy and correlation with age, sex and sorineural involvement. *Otolaryngol Neurotol*. 2002;23:431–438.

Bornemann C, Bornemann H, Franke KD, et al. Tympanocochleare Szintigraphie bei Otosklerose. *Arch Otorhinolaryngol*. 1982;235:499–500.

Bornemann H, Hundeshagen H, Franke KD. Digitale Szintigraphie des Ohres. *Arch Ohr Nas Kehlk Heilk*. 1981;231:689–691.

Chole RA, McKenna M. Pathophysiology of otosclerosis. *Otolaryngol Neurotol*. 2001; 22:249–257.

Guneri EA, Ada E, Ceryan K, et al. High resolution computed tomographic evaluation of the otic capsule in otosclerosis: relationship between densitometry and sensorineural hearing loss. *Ann Otol, Rhinol Laryngol*. 1996;105:659–664.

Huizing EH, de Groot JA. Densitometry of the otic capsule and correlation between bone density loss and bone conduction hearing loss in otosclerosis. *Acta Otolaryngol*. 1987;103:464–468.

Mafee MF, Henrikson GC, Deitch RL, et al. Use of CT in stapedial otosclerosis. *Radiology*. 1985;156:709–714.

Mafee MF, Valvassori GE, Deitch RL, et al. Use of CT in cochlear otosclerosis. *Radiology*. 1985;156:703–708.

Miura M, Naito Y, Takahashi H, et al. Computed tomographic image analysis of ears with otosclerosis. *ORL*. 1996;58:200–203.

Nager GT. Histopathology of otoscelerosis. *Arch Otolaryn*gol. 1969;89:157–159.

Ross UH, Laszig R, Bornemann H, et al. Osteogenesis imperfecta: Clinical symptoms and update findings in computed tomography and tympanocochlear scintigraphy. *Acta Otolaryngol*. 1993;113:620–624.

Ross UH, Reinhardt MJ, Reuland P. Experimental topographic study of high resolution tympanocochlear scintigraphy using the human temporal bone model. *Eur Arch Otorhinolaryngol*. 1996;53:17–20.

Ross UH, Trinhardt MJ, Berlis A. Localization of active otosclerotic foci by tympanocochlear scintigraphy (TCS) using correlative imaging. *J Laryngol Otolaryngol*. 1995;109:1051–1056.

Ruckenstein MJ, Rafter KO, Montes M, Bigelow DC. Management of far advanced otosclerosis in the era of cochlear implantation. *Otolaryngol Neurotol*. 2001;22: 471–474.

Sakai O, Curtin HD, Fujita A. Otosclerosis: Computed tomography and magnetic resonance findings. *Am J Otolaryngol*. 2000;21:116–118.

Shin YJ, Calvas P, Deguine O, Charlet JP, Cognard C, Fraysse B. Correlations between computed tomography findings and family history in otosclerotic patients. *Otolaryngol Neurotol*. 2001;22:461–464.

Shin YJ, Deguine O, Sevely A, et al. Pure sensorineural hearing loss and otosclerosis: An imaging case report. *Rev Laryngol Otol Rhinol (Bord)*. 2000;121:45–47.

Shin YJ, Fraysse B, Deguine O, Cognard C, Charlet JP, Sevely A. Sensorineural hearing loss and otosclerosis: A clinical and radiologic survey of 437 cases. *Acta Otolaryngol*. 2001;12(2):200–204.

Swartz JD, Faerber EN, Wolfson RJ, et al. Fenestral otosclerosis: Significance of preoperative CT evaluation. *Radiol*. 1984;151:703–707.

Swartz JD, Ric Harnsberger H. The otic capsule and otodystrophies. In: *Imaging of the Temporal Bone*. 2nd ed. New York: Thieme; 1992:192–246.

Syms MJ, Petermann GW. Magnetic resonance imaging of stapes prostheses. *Am J Otolaryngol*. 2000;21:494–498.

Thiers FA, Valvasorri GE, Nadol JB. Otosclerosis of the cochlear capsule: Correlation of computerized tomography and histopathology. *Am J Otolaryngol*. 1999;20:93–95.

Valvassori GE. The interpretation of the radiographic findings in cochlear otosclerosis. *Ann Otolaryngol, Rhinol Laryngol*. 1966;75:572–578.

Valvassori GE. Cochlear aqueduct by polytomography. In: *Proceedings of the Fifth International Workshop on Middle Ear Microsurgery in Fluctuant Hearing Loss*. Huntsville, AL: Strobe; 1977:565–566.

Valvasorri GE. Imaging of otosclerosis. *Otolaryngol Clin N Am*. 1993;26:359–371.

Ziheh S, Berlis A, Ross UH, et al. MRI of active otosclerosis. *Neuroradiol*. 1997;39:453–457.

# Chapter 6

# Cochlear Otosclerosis

*Cochlear otosclerosis* is a controversial term. Some authors prefer the lengthy term *sensorineural hearing loss associated with otosclerosis* because the cause-and-effect relationship is unclear. There has also been a lack of definite evidence and an associated lack of comprehensive studies of cochlear otosclerosis. For clarity, we refer to cochlear otosclerosis in this book.

## DEFINITION

Cochlear otosclerosis is a gradually progressive sensorineural hearing loss caused by the direct or indirect enzymatic action of the otosclerotic microfoci in the otic capsule. The sensorineural hearing loss is usually bilateral and symmetrical, and, as in stapedial otosclerosis, it may undergo periods of activation and remission. Pure tone and speech audiometry usually shows either a pure sensorineural hearing loss or a mixed type hearing loss.

## INCIDENCE

Pure cochlear otosclerosis without stapedial involvement is a difficult condition to identify. The incidence of cochlear otosclerosis is greater than is generally believed. In a double-blind study on histologic and polytomographic correlations in cochlear otosclerosis, Linthicum et al (1981) found that two thirds of cases had cochlear otosclerosis. The clinical incidence of cochlear otosclerosis, however, is much more difficult to determine. Freeman (1979) compared clinical and polytomographic data in 100 consecutive cases of progressive sensorineural hearing loss and found that 29% of cochlear otosclerosis cases that were suspected on clinical grounds were confirmed by polytomography. Causse and Causse (1991), in an evaluation of 11,062 cases, found a similar percentage of cases (22.9%) suffered from cochlear otosclerosis. They believed that this percentage would have been higher if polytomography had been used systematically. They stated further that the incidence of cochlear otosclerosis in progressive sensorineural hearing loss occurs frequently enough to warrant that such patients be thoroughly evaluated to eliminate the possibility of cochlear otosclerosis. Females are more affected than males, and the age of onset is similar to that of stapedial oto-sclerosis.

The clinical development of cochlear otosclerosis depends on the progression of otosclerotic focus. This in turn depends on other factors such as the genetic predisposition of the patient and endocrine factors such as puberty and pregnancy. Because the progress of cochlear otosclerosis depends on wide-ranging factors, the disease process itself undergoes periods of activation and periods of remission.

## SIGNS AND SYMPTOMS

In cases of cochlear otosclerosis, there is usually a dominant family history; the patient usually has relatives who have suffered from proven otosclerosis. The hearing loss may have started or increased during pregnancy or following the use of oral contraceptives. Examination of the tympanic membrane frequently demonstrates a positive Schwartze's sign. Apart from a sensorineural hearing loss, which is the sine qua non of cochlear otosclerosis, the patient usually experiences tinnitus and vertigo.

## SPECIALIZED HEARING TESTS

The most common pattern of pure tone audiogram is the "cookie bite" (see Chapter 4, Fig. 4–1). In cochlear otosclerosis, the audiological pattern is one of end organ disease. The Békésey audiogram is usually a type 2. There is a moderate tone decay of up to 20 dB. Speech discrimination scores of 80 to 90% are typical of cochlear otosclerosis. The short increment sensitivity index (SISI) scores are high (60 to 100%), and loudness discomfort may be present at 10 to 110 dB. The stapedial reflex is usually present (Morrison 1984).

## TINNITUS

Although tinnitus is present in stapedial otosclerosis, the incidence at which it occurs in cochlear otosclerosis is higher. It is encountered in the older age group, especially when combined otosclerosis is present. In pure cochlear otosclerosis, tinnitus is usually the presenting symptom.

## VERTIGO

Endolymphatic hydrops is commonly seen as a complication of cochlear otosclerosis. Benign paroxysmal positional vertigo is also commonly seen. Transient episodes of positional vertigo were commonly seen in about 20% of patients suffering from cochlear otosclerosis, and symptoms of hydrops were seen in about 6% of patients (Morrison 1984).

In some cases, there can be little doubt about making a diagnosis of cochlear otosclerosis, whereas in others the diagnosis may not be so apparent. In order to help make an accurate diagnosis with the intent to treat promptly with the appropriate modality, many authors have proposed several criteria with which a diagnosis of cochlear otosclerosis can be made. These criteria are as follows.

## DIAGNOSING COCHLEAR OTOSCLEROSIS

Shambaugh and Holdermann (1926) stated that for a patient to be labeled as suffering from otosclerosis, three criteria should be satisfied:

1. Insidious onset of hearing loss in early adulthood

2. The absence of any other cause that could be proven to have caused hearing loss

3. Conductive deafness in other members of the immediate family

In 1966, Shambaugh delineated six criteria for making a diagnosis of cochlear otosclerosis:

1. A positive Schwartze's sign

2. A family history of confirmed and surgically proven otosclerosis

3. The presence of symmetrical sensorineural hearing loss in both ears accompanied by stapes fixation

4. A flat, rising, or "cookie bite" audiogram with unusually good speech discrimination for a sensorineural hearing loss

5. Pure sensorineural hearing loss that begins insidiously in early life, which cannot be demonstrated to have arisen from any other cause

6. Fixation of the stapes in a patient with sensorineural hearing loss

Beales (1981) suggested eight parameters that help identify the patient suffering from cochlear otosclerosis:

1. Sensorineural hearing loss with very good speech discrimination

2. Recruitment present; high SISI scores with a Békésy type 2 audiogram

3. Progression of a sensorineural hearing loss from early adulthood

4. Bilateral and symmetrical sensorineural hearing loss

5. Unusual in configuration in the audiogram

6. Patient history of successful use of a hearing aid before the hearing loss progresses to a severe degree

7. Paracusis of Willis in the early history of the deafness

8. A negative Rinne test

Causse et al (1975) described three types of criteria for making a diagnosis of cochlear otosclerosis:

1. Criteria of presumption

   a. Slow progressive sensorineural hearing loss since childhood that becomes aggravated at puberty. There should be a family history of progressive sensorineural hearing loss.

    **b.** Sensorineural hearing loss in women is aggravated by pregnancy, menstruation, menopause, or following the use of oral contraceptives or following treatment with estrogens.

    **c.** The patient using a hearing aid should have good speech discrimination and a sensorineural hearing loss, especially during simultaneous conversation or in noisy surroundings.

**2.** Criteria for probability

    **a.** A positive Schwartze's sign should be present in one or both ears.

    **b.** A sensorineural hearing loss is detected with a "cookie bite" audiogram.

    **c.** Positive findings are seen on radiological imaging for otosclerosis (see Chapter 2, Fig. 2–2B).

**3.** Criteria of certainty

    **a.** The appearance of an "on-off" impedance effect (diphasic impedance change) is found, indicating impending fixation of the stapes in a case of slowly progressive pure sensorineural hearing loss.

    **b.** An air-bone gap (even a small one) in one ear is seen in a case of slowly progressive symmetrical pure sensorineural hearing loss and the replacement of the on-off effect by the disappearance of the stapedius reflex.

    **c.** CT densitometry demonstrates cochlear otosclerosis.

## HISTOPATHOLOGICAL CORRELATES

Lindsay and Beal (1966) found sensorineural hearing losses in temporal bones with extensive and multifocal otosclerosis. Elonka and Applebaum (1981) found an increase in bone conduction levels only in ears with two or more sites of endosteal involvement. Schuknecht and Barber (1985) found no correlation between the magnitude of sensorineural hearing loss and endosteal involvement or the size, activity, and location of the otosclerotic focus (Fig 6–1). Linthicum (1967), however, demonstrated a relationship between the degree of cochlear endosteal involvement and the hyalinization of the spiral ligament and sensorineural hearing loss. Hueb and Goycoolea (1991) in their study found that the otosclerotic focus expands from the anterior margin of the oval window toward the apex of the cochlea and involves the endosteum of the upper half of the basal turns, sometimes without stapedial fixation. Cochlear otosclerosis can occur without stapedial fixation, although any otosclerotic focus large enough to cause sensorineural hearing loss invariably causes stapedial fixation. The authors also note that in cochlear otosclerosis, the cochlea endosteum was involved only in the area of the basal turn, sometimes with atrophy and hyalinization of the spiral ligament and atrophy of the stria vascularis. Johnsson et al (1978) noted that this area of the basal turn becomes a target for possible toxic substances released by the otosclerotic focus, which results in sensorineural hearing loss when it involves the endosteum of the scalae, especially when the lesion is active.

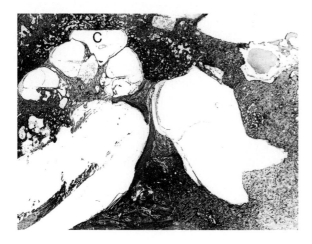

**Figure 6–1** Photomicrograph of a human temporal bone with cochlear otosclerosis. The otosclerotic focus has enveloped and deformed the cochlea (C).

## MECHANISMS BY WHICH SENSORINEURAL HEARING LOSS IS THOUGHT TO OCCUR IN COCHLEAR OTOSCLEROSIS

Toxic metabolites are thought to be liberated by the active otosclerotic focus into the inner ear fluids (Nager 1969). Chevance et al (1970) and Causse and Chevance (1978) demonstrated the presence of proteolytic enzymes in the perilymph.

Vascular compromise and hypoxic lesions of the structures of the inner ear were proposed by Ruedi (1969). He demonstrated the presence of venous shunts between the otosclerotic focus and the vessels of the inner ear that caused venous congestion, which resulted in hypoxia of the cochlea.

## RADIOLOGICAL DEMONSTRATION OF COCHLEAR OTOSCLEROSIS

Conventional radiography is of little value in otosclerosis, especially in the case of cochlear otosclerosis. Linear tomography is similarly of limited value. CT scanning is the only imaging modality that is of some value in otosclerosis. For the otosclerosis focus to be picked up on CT scanning, the focus has to be bigger than 1 mm. The otic capsule bone is the densest bone in the body and cannot become more dense. It can, however, increase in thickness. Thus, otosclerotic deposits can be picked up in the inactive phase. In the active phase, when bone resorption occurs, the otic capsule appears roughened or scalloped, its outlines becoming irregular. Derlacki and Valvassori (1965) demonstrated that otic capsule changes can be seen in 65% of patients with fenestral otosclerosis and in 30% of patients in whom cochlear otosclerosis has been suspected.

## TREATMENT OF COCHLEAR OTOSCLEROSIS

There have been numerous publications on the efficacy of sodium fluoride in the treatment of cochlear otosclerosis (Ramsay and Linthicum 1994). All claim to have arrested the progress of sensorineural hearing loss. In a study by Derks et al (2001), CT scanning and audiometric evaluation were used to monitor the progress of 19 patients treated with fluoride for 1 to 5 years and were matched with 22 untreated controls. The researchers found that fluoride was more effective for higher frequencies in cases of sensorineural hearing loss of less than 50 dB. They also found that fluoride treatment for 4 years did not seem to be superior to a shorter treatment. They noted that CT scanning did not provide reliable information as to the efficacy of fluoride treatment. Hearing loss stabilized and did not progress during treatment. Once treatment was stopped, however, six patients experienced minimal deterioration in sensorineural hearing loss. The medical management of cochlear otosclerosis includes sodium fluoride in association with calcium, vitamin D, and diphosphonates.

## ROLE OF SURGERY IN PATIENTS SUFFERING FROM COCHLEAR OTOSCLEROSIS

Surgery may be useful for those patients presenting with a hearing loss so profound that bone threshold cannot be evaluated and a gap between air and bone conduction cannot be excluded. In such circumstances, stapes surgery can improve hearing to a level that may provide a useful application for a hearing aid. It should be remembered that, to be effective, surgery must be combined with the administration of sodium fluoride.

## SUMMARY

Cochlear otosclerosis is a controversial entity. Treatment consists mainly of sodium fluoride, calcium, vitamin D, and diphosphonates. Surgery can be useful in certain situations and serves to permit benefits from amplification from a hearing aid.

## REFERENCES

Beales PH. Diagnosis of sensorineural deafness. In: *Otosclerosis*. Bristol: John Wright and Sons; 1981:68–75.

Causse JR, Causse JB. Prognosis: Sensorineural deterioration and cochlear otosclerosis. In: *Otosclerosis (otospongiosis)*. Alexandria, Va.: American Academy of Otolaryngology—Head and Neck Surgery Foundation Inc.:87–96.

Causse JR, Chevance LG. Sensorineural hearing loss due to cochlear otospongiosis: etiology. *Otolaryngol Clin N Am*. 1978;11:125–134.

Causse J, Shambaugh GE, Chevance LG, Bretlau P. Cochlear otospongiosis: etiology, diagnosis and therapeutic implications. *Ann Otorhinolaryngol*. 1975;22:43–47.

Chevance L, Jorgensen MB, Bretlau P, Causse J. Electron microscopic studies of the otosclerotic focus. *Acta Otolaryngol*. 1970;67:563–568.

Derks W, de Groot JA, Raymakers JA, Veldmann JE. Fluoride therapy for cochlear otosclerosis: An audiometric and computerized tomography evaluation. *Acta Otolaryngol*. 2001;121:174–177.

Derlacki E, Valvassori G. Clinical and radiological diagnosis of labyrinthine otosclerosis. *Laryngoscope*. 1965;75:1293–1306.

Elonka DR, Applebaum EL. Otosclerotic involvement in the cochlea: A histologic and audiologic study. *Otolaryngol Head Neck Surg*. 1981;89:343–351.

Freeman J. Progressive sensorineural hearing loss and cochlear otosclerosis: A prospective study. *Laryngoscope*. 1979;89:1487–1521.

Hueb MM, Goycoolea MV. The University of Minnesota Temporal Bone Collection. *Otolaryngol Head Neck Surg.* 1991;105:396–405.

Johnsson LG, Hawkins JE, Linthicum FH. Cochlear and vestibular lesions in capsular otosclerosis as seen in microdissection. *Ann Otol Rhinol Laryngol.* 1978;87(suppl 48):1–40.

Lindsay JR, Beal DD. Sensorineural deafness in otosclerosis: Observations on histopathology. *Ann Otol Rhinol Laryngol.* 1966;75:436–457.

Linthicum FH. Pathology and pathogenesis of sensorineural deafness. *ENT Digest.* 1967;29:51–56.

Linthicum FH, Ruenas R, Belal A. Histologic and polytomographic correlation in cochlear otosclerosis. In: Shambaugh GE Jr, Shea JJ, eds. *Shambaugh-Shea International Workshop on Microsurgery.* Huntsville, Ala.: Strode; 1981:468–471.

Morrison AW. Diseases of the otic capsule: Otosclerosis. In: Ballantyne JC, Groves J, Scott-Brown WG, eds. *Scott-Brown's Diseases of the Ear, Nose and Throat.* 4th ed. Boston: Butterworth World Student Reprints; 1979:405–464.

Nager GT. Histopathology of otosclerosis. *Acta Otolaryngol.* 1969;89:341–362.

Ramsay HA, Linthicum FH. Mixed hearing loss in otosclerosis: Indication for long term follow-up. *Am J Otol.* 1994;15:536–539.

Ruedi L. Otosclerotic lesions and cochlear degeneration. *Arch Otolaryngol.* 1969;78:469–473.

Schuknecht H, Barber W. Histologic variants in otosclerosis. *Laryngoscope.* 1985;95:1307–1317.

Shambaugh GE. Therapy of otosclerosis. *Ann Otolaryngol.* 1966;75:579–583.

Shambaugh GE, Holderman JW. The occurrence of otosclerosis in the aetiology of progressive deafness. *Arch Otolaryngol.* 1926;4:127–129.

# Chapter 7

# Medical Treatment of Otosclerosis

Any treatment that can arrest the progression of deafness in cochlear or combined otosclerosis must be given serious consideration. Even those who deny the very existence of cochlear otosclerosis admit that mixed deafness can occur in otosclerosis and can have devastating consequences. This cannot be remedied by surgery alone. Thus, alternative therapies need to be considered for these situations, especially in arresting the progress of sensorineural hearing loss associated with otosclerosis.

Shambaugh and Scott (1964) first suggested that sodium fluoride in moderate dosages could promote recalcification and reduce bone resorption in an active otosclerotic focus. In another study, Petrovic and Shambaugh (1966) reported the effects of this treatment on laboratory animals. They found that sodium fluoride accelerates the calcification of bone and the healing of fractures by inducing speedy formation of a callus and slowing down the decalcification that precedes the healing of fractures.

In humans, fluoride is very effective on the active otosclerotic focus, although it is not that effective on an inactive focus. It was found in vitro that otosclerotic lesions take up radioactive calcium much more readily if fluoride is added to the culture medium.

Sodium fluoride is a trace substance found naturally in varying concentrations (between 0.1 and 16 parts per million) in ground water. Some local authorities add fluoride to drinking water to increase the concentration to 1 part per million, and this has proven very effective in preventing cavities in teeth.

Bernstein et al (1966) examined rural communities in North Dakota and found that there was an abnormally low fluoride content in the drinking water, which was accompanied by a high incidence of osteoporosis. Daniel (1969) compared the incidence of stapedial fixation in an area of low fluoride concentration with that in an area of high fluoride concentration in the drinking water. He found that stapedial fixation was four times higher in the low fluoride concentration than in the high fluoride concentration. Petrovic and Shambaugh (1966) demonstrated in animal studies that with an optimum dose of fluoride bone resorption decreases and calcification increases. They also indicated that their dosages were very minimal, well below the minimum lethal dosage, thereby indicating that sodium fluoride is a very safe drug in therapeutic dosages.

## HOW DOES SODIUM FLUORIDE ACT?

Fluorides act by reducing bone resorption and increasing osteoblastic bone formation. Causse et al (1973) postulated that in otosclerosis fluorides have an antienzymatic action on proteolytic enzymes that are cytotoxic to the cochlea. Sodium fluoride is effective only when the otosclerotic focus is active. Sodium fluoride reduces osteoclastic bone resorption and at the same time promotes osteoblastic bone formation. In new bone the fluoride ion replaces the hydroxy radical in hydroxyapatite; the resulting fluorapatite is harder, of better quality, and more resistant to bone resorption than hydroxyapatite.

Sodium fluoride in optimum dosages accelerates the healing of fractures by hastening the calcification of the callus formation. Fluoride prevents cortisone-induced osteoporosis. It also promotes maturation of active otosclerosis by reducing vascularity and bone resorption activity and by increasing new bone formation to eventually produce inactive otosclerosis. Petrovic and Shambaugh (1966) found that acid phenylphosphatase, the enzyme of bone resorption, is markedly elevated in organ cultures of active otosclerosis. After short-term sodium fluoride therapy of 6 months, the enzyme begins to decline. After long-term fluoride therapy, the enzyme was found to decline to low levels. Petrovic and Shambaugh (1966) measured the uptake of radioactive calcium in organ cultures and discovered it to be increased by spongiotic (active otosclerotic focus) bone. Following short-term fluoride therapy, they noted a significant additional increase of calcium uptake as bone deposition is stimulated. After fluoride therapy for more than 1 year, the calcium uptake was found to decline markedly to that found in inactive otosclerosis. It must be noted that in all of Petrovic and Shambaugh's work, the dose of fluoride was critical; the optimum dosage used in adults was 60 mg daily.

## RATIONALE FOR THE USE OF SODIUM FLUORIDE IN OTOSCLEROSIS

The rationale for the use of sodium fluoride for the treatment of cochlear or combined otosclerosis is based on the following evidence in the literature. Daniel (1969) demonstrated that there is an increase of stapedial otosclerosis in areas where the levels of fluoride were low. Petrovic and Shambaugh (1966) demonstrated in young rats that sodium fluoride in optimum doses promoted new bone formation and reduced bone resorption. The rationale also follows reports that changes occur in the clinical and radiological conditions of patients suffering from cochlear or combined otosclerosis when sodium fluoride is administered.

Causse and colleagues (1993) found that sodium fluoride influences underlying bony changes in the labyrinth so as to arrest or prevent the onset of hearing loss. Sodium fluoride is an enzyme inhibitor, reduces osteoclastic bone resorption, and, if the dosage is more than 60 mg a day, may rebuild pseudohaversian bone.

## CLINICAL DATA ON THE EFFECTIVENESS OF SODIUM FLUORIDE

Bretlau et al (1985) conducted a double-blind trial to determine the effectiveness of fluoride on otosclerosis. Using a calcium to phosphate ratio as an indication of bone maturity, they judged the efficacy of fluoride in stabilizing otosclerosis by the retention of calcium levels relative to phosphorus. The clinical double-blind placebo-controlled study of 95 patients showed a statistically significant worse deterioration of the hearing loss in the placebo group than in the active treated group (40 mg sodium fluoride daily). Bretlau et al found that fluoride can change otospongiotic active lesions to more dense inactive otosclerotic lesions.

Causse and colleagues (1981, 1982) presented their findings from 648 perilymph samples taken during stapedectomies performed from February 1976 through September 1980. They studied microdosages of three selected enzymes: trypsin, alpha$_1$-antitrypsin, and alpha$_2$-macroglobulin; in each of the samples, the enzymes' relationship with cochlear deterioration expressed in decibels of bone conduction decreased in pure tone audiometry testing. The authors discovered that fluoride not only inhibits direct trypsin inhibition but also results in an overall reduction in enzymatic values in the perilymph of otosclerotic patients.

## INDICATIONS FOR THE USE OF SODIUM FLUORIDE

Sodium fluoride can be administered under the following circumstances:

1. Patients with surgically confirmed otosclerosis who demonstrate progressive sensorineural deafness disproportionate to age

2. Patients who present with sensorineural deafness (cochlear otosclerosis). These patients should have a family history of otosclerosis. Their age of onset should be early, with an audiometric pattern suggestive of otosclerosis. They should also have good speech discrimination. Forquer et al (1986) examined the effectiveness of fluoride in the treatment of cochlear otosclerosis in 94 patients with cochlear otosclerosis and 98 patients with stapedial otosclerosis and sensorineural hearing loss. Fluoride halted or slowed the progression of sensorineural hearing loss in 63% of patients with cochlear otosclerosis and 46% of patients with stapedial otosclerosis. In their study, the single factor that predicted which patients would respond most favorably to treatment was rate of progression before treatment. Fluoride therapy was successful for 79% of the patients losing their hearing at a rate of 5 dB or more per year at one or more of the speech frequencies. The researchers thus concluded that patients with more rapid rates of progression responded most favorably to fluoride therapy. In other words, the most active otosclerotic lesion responded the most to fluoride.

3. Patients with radiological changes compatible with those of otosclerosis

4. Patients with a positive Schwartze's sign

5. Patients who have otosclerosis and also are diagnosed to present with secondary hydrops

6. Stapedial otosclerosis, without sensorineural hearing loss, when surgery has been refused by the patient and the patient seeks alternative forms of treatment

Colletti and Fiorino (1991) presented the effectiveness of fluoride treatment in modifying the natural course of subclinical otosclerosis. They used the stapedial reflex as a parameter by which they could measure the response and effectiveness of treatment. The diagnosis of subclinical otosclerosis was made on the basis of the presence of the on-off effect of the stapedial reflex. The study was carried out on 128 relatives of patients suffering from surgically confirmed otosclerosis. One group of patients was treated with sodium fluoride in doses ranging from 6 to 16 mg according to age for a period of 2 years. The second group served as a control. Changes in stapedius reflex morphology were evaluated at 1, 2, and 5 years from the onset of treatment. The investigation demonstrated that fluoride has a stabilizing effect on early otosclerosis. They reported that fluoride arrests the disease process in more than 60% of ears at the 2-year follow-up and in more than 50% at 5 years. On the basis of this report, the authors suggested a program of secondary prevention of otosclerosis.

## CONTRAINDICATIONS TO SODIUM FLUORIDE THERAPY

Sodium fluoride is contraindicated in the following situations:

1. Patients who have chronic nephritis with nitrogen retention should not receive fluorides. In such circumstances, they might not be able to excrete fluoride, leading to a toxic buildup.

2. Patients who suffer from chronic rheumatoid arthritis. During initial therapy, patients suffering from chronic rheumatoid arthritis experience an increase in joint pains. However, these subside after a few weeks of treatment.

3. Those patients who are pregnant or lactating should not receive sodium fluoride. The effects of sodium fluoride on the fetus and the newborn are unknown.

4. Children in whom skeletal growth has not yet been achieved should not receive sodium fluoride.

5. Patients with skeletal fluorosis must be excluded. This is a rare condition in which skeletal fluorosis occurs due to high (toxic) levels of fluoride in drinking water.

6. Those patients who have an allergy to fluoride will obviously be excluded from receiving this drug.

## DOSAGE AND ADMINISTRATION OF SODIUM FLUORIDE

When an active otosclerotic lesion is thought to be present, a daily dose of 50 mg of sodium fluoride is given. If the lesion is present with Schwartze's sign, and a sensorineural component is present, then the dose may be increased to 75 mg daily. When the hearing stabilizes, Schwartze's sign fades, and there is radiological evidence of recalcification, then a maintenance dose of 25 mg may be given for the rest of the patient's life.

Fluorical, used as a dietary supplement in the United States, contains 8.3 mg of sodium fluoride and 364 mg of calcium carbonate per capsule. Two capsules of Fluorical taken three times a day will supply approximately 50 mg of sodium fluoride, with 2184 mg of calcium carbonate—sufficient to provide the calcium needed for the new bone formation that the sodium fluoride has induced. Four hundred units of vitamin D should also be given from time to time to ensure intestinal absorption of the calcium.

Side effects can occur with fluoride; their frequency is comparable to the frequency of the side effects of aspirin. Sodium fluoride has been used since 1960 for the treatment of osteoporosis and has been given to over 20,000 patients without a single instance of permanent harm (Beales 1981). Note that a single dose of about 5 g or more can be fatal (Shambaugh and Wiet 1980).

## RESULTS OF TREATMENT WITH SODIUM FLUORIDE

### Hearing Loss Stabilized

Shambaugh and Causse (1974) reported the results of treatment with sodium fluoride in over 4000 patients. Eighty percent of patients who had a sensorineural hearing loss had their hearing stabilized. The remaining patients continued to experience a slow progression of the hearing loss. This study included a smaller control group who did not receive treatment. This group experienced a more rapid progression of hearing loss than those who received treatment with sodium fluoride but whose hearing did not stabilize.

Derks et al (2001) published a report on the progress of sensorineural hearing loss (SNHL) in patients with cochlear otosclerosis. Nineteen patients suffering from cochlear otosclerosis were treated with fluoride for 1 to 5 years and were compared with 22 controls. CT scans of eight patients before and after treatment with fluoride were evaluated. The authors reported that fluoride therapy arrested the progression of SNHL in the low (250 Hz, 500 Hz, and 1 kHz) ($p = 0.001$) and high (2 and 4 kHz) ($p = .008$) frequencies. It seemed to be more effective for the higher frequencies in cases with an initial SNHL of 50 dB. Fluoride administration for 4 years did not seem to be superior to a shorter treatment period (1 to 2 years). Six patients were followed up after discontinuing fluoride therapy, and even they showed minimal deterioration in SNHL.

Ramsay and Linthicum (1994) published a retrospective study of 146 ears with long-term follow-up after otosclerosis surgery to evaluate the stability of hearing results, the incidence of sensorineural hearing loss, and the effect of fluoride therapy. Follow-up was for a period of 15 years (mean 25.2 years; range 15 to 44 years). There were 97 large fenestra surgeries, 23 lateral canal fenestrations, 7 mobilizations, and 19 revision stapes surgeries. Sodium fluoride was used to treat 11 ears with progressive sensorineural hearing loss. The rate of bone conduction hearing deterioration decreased in all ears after treatment, and none developed profound sensorineural hearing loss. Ramsay and Linthicum thus concluded their report by recommending sodium fluoride for patients who have sensorineural hearing loss as the result of otosclerosis.

Clinical proof of the effectiveness of fluoride in optimum dosage to promote maturation of active otosclerosis (converting an active otosclerotic focus to an inactive focus) has been demonstrated by Linthicum et al (1973). Shambaugh and Causse (1974) and Causse et al (1974) demonstrated in a case-controlled study of 575 patients that 80% of these patients when treated with fluoride exhibited stabilization of their sensorineural hearing loss. The patients' hearing stabilized, and they did not exhibit further deterioration in hearing. Another 3% of these patients demonstrated an improvement in hearing, and 17% experienced deterioration in hearing despite receiving fluoride. In 8%, sensorineural hearing loss started when the sodium fluoride was stopped.

Several double-blind prospective studies (Bretlau et al 1985; Bretlau et al 1989; Fisch 1985) confirmed that sodium fluoride does stabilize hearing in sensorineural hearing loss, while the controls who do not receive treatment continue to experience a deterioration in their hearing. Vartiainen and Vartiainen (1996) reported significantly improved bone conduction thresholds at 2 and 4 kHz in ears that had previously undergone stapedectomy.

## Stapedial Reflex

In a study conducted by Colletti and Fiorino (1987), the stapedial reflex was evaluated in 93 relatives of those patients suffering from otosclerosis that was confirmed surgically. The subjects were divided into two groups, the first group being treated with sodium fluoride for 2 years. The second group served as controls. Before the start of the study, all subjects (groups 1 and 2) had abnormalities in the reflex morphology as evidenced by a partial to complete on-off effect in one or both ears. Changes in stapedial reflex morphology (from partial to complete on-off and from complete on-off to absence of the reflex) were evaluated at 1 and 2 years. Both groups did not develop significant differences at 1 year. At year 2, however, the incidence of stable stapedius reflex findings was 91.5% in the treated ears and 77% in the control group. The difference was significant ($p < .05$) and indicated the stabilizing effect of sodium fluoride on the otosclerotic disease process.

## Control of Vestibular Symptoms

Freeman (1980) demonstrated that sodium fluoride was effective not only in controlling sensorineural hearing loss but also in reversing symptoms of vestibular dysfunction.

## Radiological Evidence of Improvement

Radiological evidence of arrest of otosclerosis is not in itself sufficient evidence that otosclerosis has been arrested. Radiological evidence must be combined with audiological evidence that the progress of otosclerosis has been halted.

Other studies, however, did demonstrate that the otosclerotic focus matures with the administration of sodium fluoride.

## Enzymatic Evidence

Causse et al (1993) postulated that sodium fluoride is an enzymatic inhibitor and reduces osteoclastic bone resorption; if the dosage of sodium fluoride is more than 60 mg per day, it may build pseudohaversian bone. Small doses of sodium fluoride were effective in inhibiting protein metabolism. Fluoride was found to be essential to protect the hair cells of the labyrinth from toxic damage by the enzymes of bone resorption produced by active otosclerosis (Causse et al 1973).

## Side Effects of Sodium Fluoride Therapy

Those patients who have received sodium fluoride therapy should receive a skeletal survey that should be repeated every 2 years. Also, a skeletal survey should be done before the administration of sodium fluoride. Shambaugh (1989) observed radiological evidence of early fluorosis of the spine in 0.25% of patients. This condition is reversible when treatment is discontinued.

Gastric disturbances are a common side effect. These occur because of the production of hydrofluoric acid in the stomach. This side effect can be prevented by an enteric coating on the fluoride tablet.

Those patients suffering from chronic arthritis may experience an increase in arthralgia in their joints. This stops when treatment is stopped, however.

Beales (1981) emphasized that there was no record in the literature of permanent damage caused by sodium fluoride when used in a proper manner.

## OTHER MEDICATIONS

### Biphosphonates (Diphosphonates)

When sodium fluoride is not well tolerated, biphosphonates, also known as diphosphonates, can be given. Biphosphonates are new, promising medications that can be used in the treatment of otosclerosis. They are administered orally. Their mechanism of action is that they are incorporated into bone and inhibit osteoclastic activity. Other postulated mechanisms of action are primary enzymatic inhibition and promoting stable secondary new bone formation. Biphosphonates are well tolerated and effective. Newer biphosphonates have negligible effects on bone formation. Brookler and Tanyeri (1997) discovered that etidronate appeared to halt the progression of otosclerotic foci, as observed with high-resolution CT scanning. In this past decade, biphosphonates like etidronate and alendronate have been used widely for the treatment of osteoporosis, with well-documented beneficial effects and no accompanying adverse effects. There were a few reports (Boumans and Poublon 1991; Yasil et al 1998) that claimed sensorineural hearing loss in otosclerotic patients who were treated with the first-generation biphosphonates aminohydroxypropylidene and etidronate. However, the widespread use of alendronate has not been associated with sensorineural hearing loss. The most promising biphosphonates are those potent inhibitors of bone resorption, such as third-generation biphosphonates like alendronate, residronate, and zolendronate.

### Cytokine Inhibitors

Cytokine antagonists may suppress the resorption seen in otosclerosis. Interleukin-1 receptor antagonist and tumor necrosis factor (TNF) binding protein have been shown to halt bone resorption that invariably occurs following ovariectomy. It is thought to be quite likely that these factors inhibit bone modeling as well (Merkel et al 1999). Cytokine inhibitors are thought to be promising because it is likely that these compounds would halt the progress of otosclerosis. However, it is thought that these would be best used when the otosclerotic focus is in its active phase (Chole and McKenna 2001).

## REFERENCES

Beales PH. Medical treatment. In: *Otosclerosis*. Bristol: John Wright and Sons; 1981: 76–84.

Bernstein DS, Sadowski N, Hagstead DM. The prevalence of osteoporosis in high and low fluoride areas of North Dakota. *JAMA*. 1966;198:499.

Boumans LJ, Poublon RM. The detrimental effect of aminohydroxypropylidene biphosphonate (APD) in otospongiosis. *Euro Arch Otorhinolaryngol*. 1991;248:218–221.

Bretlau P, Causse J, Causse JB, Hansen HJ, Johnsen NJ, Salomon G. Otospongiosis and sodium fluoride: A blind experimental and clinical evaluation of the effect of sodium fluoride treatment in patients with otospongiosis. *Ann Otol, Rhinol Laryngol*. 1985;94(2, pt 1):103–107.

Bretlau P, Salomon G, Johnsen NJ. Otospongiosis and sodium fluoride: A clinical double blind placebo controlled study on sodium fluoride treatment in otospongiosis. *Am J Otol*. 1989;10(1):20–22.

Brookler KH, Tanyeri H. Etidronate for the neurotologic symptoms of otosclerosis: Preliminary study. *Ear, Nose Throat J*. 1997;76:371–376, 379–381.

Causse JR, Causse JB, Uriel J, Berges J, Shambaugh GE, Bretlau P. Sodium fluoride therapy. *Am J Otol*. 1993;14(5):482–490.

Causse JR, Chevance LG, Shambaugh GE. Clinical experience and experimental findings with sodium fluoride in otosclerosis (otospongiosis). *Ann Otol, Rhinol Laryngol*. 1974;83:643–647.

Causse JR, Chevance LG, Uriel J. Cellular and enzymatic concept of otospongiosis: Cytoclinical relationship. *Proceedings of the 10th World Congress, Venice, Italy* (Excerpta Medica International Congress Series). 1973;337:376–381.

Causse JR, Uriel J, Berges J, Shambaugh GE, Bretlau P, Causse JB. The enzymatic mechanism of the otospongiotic disease and NaF action on the enzymatic balance. *Am J Otol*. 1982;3(4):297–314.

Causse JR, Uriel J, Berges J, Bretlau P, Causse JB. Enzymatic mechanism of otosclerosis: Action of NaF. *Annales d'Oto-Laryngologie et de Chirurgie Cervico-Faciale*. 1981; 98(6):269–297.

Chole RA, McKenna M. Oathophysiology of Otosclerosis. *Otol Neurotol*. 2001;22(2) 249–257.

Colletti V, Fiorino FG. Stapedius reflex in the monitoring of NaF treatment of subclinical otosclerosis. *Acta Otolaryngol*. 1987;104(5–6):447–453.

Colletti V, Fiorino FG. Effect of sodium fluoride on early stages of otosclerosis. *Am J Otol*. 1991;12(3):195–198.

Daniel HJ. Stapedial otosclerosis and fluorine in the drinking water. *Arch Otolaryngol*. 1969;90:585.

Derks W, De Groot JA, Raymakers JA, Veldman JE. Fluoride therapy for cochlear otosclerosis: An audiometic and computerized tomography evaluation. *Acta Otolaryngol*. 2001;121(2):174–177.

Fisch U. New dimensions in the management of otosclerosis. In: *Proceedings of the 13th World Congress of Otolaryngology*. 1985:33–38.

Forquer BD, Linthicum FH, Bennett C. Sodium fluoride: Effectiveness of treatment for cochlear otosclerosis. *Am J Otol*. 1986;7(2):121–125.

Freeman J. Otosclerosis and vestibular dysfunction. *Laryngoscope*. 1980;90(9): 1481–1487.

Linthicum FH, House HO, Althous SR. The effect of sodium fluoride on otosclerotic activity as determined by strontium 85. *Trans Am Otol Soc*. 1973;61:98.

Merkel KD, Erdmann JM, McHugh KP, et al. Tumor necrosis factor alpha mediates orthopedic implant osteolysis. *Am J Pathol*. 1999;154:203–210.

Petrovic A, Shambaugh GE. A study of the effects of fluoride on bone in laboratory animals and on the otosclerotic bone in human subjects. *Arch Otolaryngol*. 1966; 83:104.

Ramsay HA, Linthicum FH. Mixed hearing loss in otosclerosis: Indication for long term follow-up. *Am J Otol*. 1994;15(4):536–539.

Shambaugh GE, Scott A. Sodium fluoride for the arrest of otosclerosis. *Arch Otolaryngol*. 1964;80:263.

Shambaugh GE, Causse JR. Ten years experience with fluoride in otosclerotic (otospongiotic) patients. *Ann Otol, Rhinol Laryngol*. 1974;83:635.

Shambaugh GE Jr, Sundan VS. Experiments and experiences with sodium fluoride for inactivation of the otosclerotic lesions. *Laryngoscope*. 1969;79:1754–1766.

Shambaugh GE Jr, Wiet JR. The fluoride treatment of otospongiosis (otosclerosis). *Can Med J*. 1980;8:29–33.

Vartiainen E, Vartiainen J. The effect of drinking water fluoridation on the natural course of hearing in patients with otosclerosis. *Acta Otolaryngol*. 1996;116:747–750.

Yasil S, Comlekci A, Guneri A. Further hearing loss during osteoporosis treatment with etidronate. *Postgrad Med J*. 1998;74:363–364.

# Chapter *8*

## Hearing Aids and Otosclerosis

Patients suffering from otosclerosis usually have a conductive hearing loss with good bone conduction, as well as excellent speech discrimination scores. Such patients with conductive-type hearing losses show excellent benefit from amplification of sound.

How severe should a conductive hearing loss be and still be classified as a purely conductive hearing loss? Reger (1940) indicated that for a hearing loss to be purely conductive, it could attain a maximum gap of 60 dB. Beyond that, he concluded, a sensorineural component was inevitable. Pohlman (1943) published a report on 10 patients who had undergone complete removal of all middle ear structures. Those patients averaged a pure conductive hearing loss of 58 dB.

### SITUATIONS APPROPRIATE FOR HEARING AIDS

Most patients with otosclerosis have severe conductive hearing losses that are accompanied by a sensorineural component. Typically, patients have a good to excellent speech discrimination score despite the severity of the conductive hearing loss.

Amplification via hearing aids or assistive listening devices must be presented to patients as viable alternatives to surgery (Johnson 1993). Not only are there medicolegal responsibilities in presenting these alternatives, but there are also many patients who may be adequately managed with amplification. Situations that are appropriate for hearing aids include the following:

1. Patient cannot undergo surgery because of major systemic illnesses.

2. Only hearing ear

3. Patient has inadequate hearing reserve and/or poor speech discrimination score.

4. Congenital fixation of the stapes is present, with the real risk of it developing into a nonhearing ear if surgery is contemplated.

5. Surgery is not elected by the patient.

6. Affected ear shows early (mild) conductive hearing loss.

7. Unsuccessful surgery for otosclerosis on the other ear has been attempted.

8. Patient has both otosclerosis and Meniere's disease.

9. Patient has stapedectomy for far-advanced otosclerosis.

It is important to assess the patient's communication needs and difficulties. It must be remembered that indications for amplification in patients with conductive hearing losses are different from candidacy criteria for those with sensorineural hearing losses because of the difference in loudness perception at comparable sensation levels. A mild conductive hearing loss may affect communication more than a mild sensorineural hearing impairment with recruitment. Patients who have a conductive hearing loss will need more amplification to achieve comfortable listening levels than those with sensorineural hearing impairment. The conductive hearing loss creates a higher tolerance for loud sounds, producing a wider dynamic range that is reflected in greater saturation sound pressure levels.

Patients suffering from otosclerosis who present with a conductive hearing loss experience paracusis of Willis. In contrast, those who have cochlear otosclerosis experience speech degradation in the presence of background noise. Such patients need less amplification in the low frequencies. Those patients who have a conductive hearing loss and otosclerosis need a well-fitting earpiece, necessary to maintain low-frequency amplification and to decrease feedback problems. Venting may not be required. The type of hearing aid will be determined by the degree and configuration of hearing loss and the patient's preference.

Audiometrically, the patients who will be the best candidates for amplification are those who do not experience distortion of the incoming speech signal and have the widest dynamic range. Theoretically, it would seem that those who suffer from otosclerosis would be ideal candidates for amplification. They will appreciate increased volume through amplification; they do not recruit to loud sounds. These factors make amplification a feasible alternative to medical or surgical modalities.

## CONTROVERSIES: HEARING AIDS OR STAPEDECTOMY

In an article that generated many rebuttals, Howard (1998) stated that hearing aids should be offered as an alternative to surgery to patients who have otosclerosis. O'Connor and Wiet (1991) stated that when presenting management alternatives to the otosclerotic patient, amplification via hearing aids or assistive listening devices or both must be offered as a viable alternative to surgical and/or medical intervention. This is necessary not only from the medicolegal point of view but also from the ethical aspect, because a significant number of patients can be managed appropriately with amplification.

Lundy (1999), in a letter to the editor responding to the article by Howard (1998), noted that his reason for advising stapedectomy over a hearing aid is because hearing aids are expensive ($800 to $2500 per hearing aid) and must be replaced every 3 to 4 years. Batteries also need to be changed every 2 weeks. In addition, repair costs must be included, which further inflates the cost of a hearing aid. Lundy further noted that hearing aids are not covered by Medicare or by the vast majority of insurers. He considers that, unless they do become a covered benefit, hearing aids are not truly an equal alternative for patients with otosclerosis.

Lundy conceded that hearing aids are essentially risk-free. In other words, they do not subject the patient to the risk of a possibly irreversible profound sensorineural hearing loss. Lundy cautioned, however, that hearing aids are not always reliable or available and that the value of treatment is more than just the risks involved.

Most of those who responded to the article by Howard (1998) conceded that the major impediment to advocating hearing aids lies in the fact that they are expensive and are not covered by Medicare or by most health insurers in the United States. Gauthier (1999), in a letter to the editor, raised the following points:

1. Stapedectomy is covered by most insurance plans, whereas hearing aids are not.

2. Would not an ethical situation demand that the patient have similar cost and benefit for both hearing aids and stapedectomy surgery?

3. Is it ethical that only the wealthy can afford the low-risk option of hearing aids?

Gianoli et al (1999) disagreed with the premise that hearing aids could be an equal alternative to a successful stapedectomy. They further noted that the quality of sound produced by a hearing aid is not equivalent to normal hearing. A successful stapedectomy patient never has trouble with acoustic feedback, never runs out of batteries, and never has to take out the hearing aid while bathing, swimming, and so on. A successful stapedectomy patient is less prone to accumulation of wax and otitis externa and has fewer problems with word discrimination in the presence of background noise.

Miller (1999), an audiologist, noted in his reply to the editor that he offers hearing aids as an alternative modality of treatment to otosclerotic patients. He favored surgery, however, when there are a large air-bone gap, good to excellent word recognition scores, and good cochlear reserve.

Finally, in his own reply to the editor, Howard (1999) conceded that hearing aids are not covered by Medicare or other insurers. This would then cause many patients to opt for surgery because stapedectomy is indeed covered by insurance.

Note that all of the authors discussed not the ethicality of the procedure but the ethics of the surgeon who will do the procedure. The questions they raised are the following:

1. Has the patient been offered amplification as an alternative modality?

Our view is that amplification must be offered as an alternative modality, not just from the aspect of compliance of medicolegal regulations but also from an ethical point of view. Everything should be placed in perspective, however. We feel that the patient should be allowed to meet and discuss with other patients who have undergone a successful stapedectomy as well as those who wear a hearing aid; this will help them appreciate the pros and cons of both modalities.

2.  What is informed consent?

Informed consent is a sine qua non of any procedure. Again, it is incumbent upon the surgeon to make it clear to the patient the real (albeit low) risk of a permanent irreversible sensorineural hearing loss that may accompany an apparently uneventful, and for all practical purposes successful, stapedectomy. This permanent irreversible sensorineural hearing loss could be immediate or delayed.

## CONCLUSIONS

The surgeon should be in a position to indicate to the patient in language that the patient can understand the complications, results, and effects of the surgery that the surgeon has encountered while performing this procedure. The figures quoted by the operating surgeon should be from the patients he or she has encountered, not from papers or books published by other surgeons.

Finally, the surgeon should be absolutely honest and should discern which patients he or she feels would genuinely benefit from amplification and those from surgery.

## REFERENCES

Gauthier MG. Never say "ever" [letter to the editor]. *Am J Otol*. 1999;20(1):138.

Gianoli GJ, Gonsoulin T, Amedee R, Tabb H, Mann W. Is stapedectomy ever ethical? Faulty premise, faulty conclusion [letter to the editor]. *Am J Otol*. 1999;20(1): 138–139.

Howard ML. Is stapedectomy ever ethical? *Am J Otol*. 1998;19:541–543.

Howard ML. Authors reply [letter to the editor]. *Am J Otol*. 1999;20(1)141.

Johnson EW. Hearing aids and otosclerosis. *Otolaryngol Clin N Am*. 1993;26:491–502.

Lundy LB. "Ethics" of stapedectomy [letter to the editor]. *Am J Otol*. 1999;20(1): 137–138.

Miller M. An audiologist replies [letter to the editor]. *Am J Otol*. 1999;20(1):140–141.

O'Connor C, Wiet RJ. Hearing aid use: An alternative to surgery. In: Wiet RJ, Causse JB, Shambaugh GE, Causse JR, eds. *Otosclerosis (Otospongiosis).* Washington, D.C.: American Academy of Otolaryngology—Head and Neck Surgery Foundation; 1991:129–133.

Pohlman AG. The diaphragm rod prosthesis of the middle ear. *Arch Otolaryngol*. 1943;37:628.

Reger S. Factors influencing the accuracy and interpretation of bone conduction and other tests. *JAMA*. 1940;11:378.

# Chapter 9

# Lasers in Otosclerosis

The use of the laser in otosclerosis was considered by Sataloff in 1967, and in 1972 by Stahle et al (1980) presented a preliminary report of argon laser stapedotomy with excellent results. DiBartolomeo and Ellis (1980) reported on the argon laser for middle ear and external ear problems, again with good results. McGee (1983) reported the use of the laser in over 100 primary stapedectomies. McGee (1989) reported shorter hospital stays, less vertigo, and excellent hearing results as the advantages of laser stapedectomies.

The single biggest advantage was the use of the laser in revision stapedectomy. For revision stapedectomy with mechanical instruments, air-bone closure to within 10 dB was achieved in fewer than half of all patients. The incidence of significant sensorineural hearing loss is 3 to 30%. The results of revision stapedectomy are significantly lower than the accepted standard for primary stapedectomy. The introduction of laser revision stapedectomy, however, has greatly improved results in terms of hearing and has reduced the incidence of permanent sensorineural hearing loss.

## LASER PHYSICS AND PRINCIPLES

The word *laser* is the acronym for light amplification by stimulated emission of radiation. Laser energy is derived from the release of photons that occurs when stimulated electrons return to their resting orbit. Albert Einstein stated that when photons of the appropriate wavelengths strike excited atoms, a second additional photon is released as the electron returns to its ground state. In this stimulated emission situation, both photons emitted from the excited atom have exactly the same frequency, direction, and phase, providing a laser beam that is collimated, coherent, and monochromatic.

Lasers differ from one another principally in the lasing medium used, which determines the wavelength of light. The energy source, along with the mechanism to excite the laser medium and release its energy, determines the mode of the laser, which is generally continuous wave (CW), pulsed, or Q switched. Q switching involves a mirror system designed to interrupt the photon emission in the lasing medium, allowing it to build to higher levels, then releasing the emission in short pulses. Delivery of the energy may be by free beam or by focused beam, or the energy may be delivered by fiber or by contact fiber tip.

Lasers typically are named for their active medium, or from the source of the atoms that are excited and undergo stimulated emission by photons. The active medium can be a solid, a liquid, or a gas. Common gas lasers are carbon dioxide, argon, and helium-neon. Solid-state lasers include neodymium:yttrium-aluminum-garnet (Nd:YAG) and the potassium titanyl phosphate (KTP) crystal. The KTP laser is an Nd:YAG laser beam that passes through a KTP crystal, which halves the wavelength (doubles the frequency) of the laser beam.

The wavelength of the laser has important characteristics for tissue interaction. Lasers whose wavelength falls in the visible spectrum (about 380 to 700 nm) and the infrared (700 nm to 1 mm) of the electromagnetic spectrum are considered thermal lasers. On contact with tissue, the laser energy is converted to thermal energy, which causes a rapid increase in tissue temperature. The laser–tissue interaction depends on the nature of the tissue (i.e., bone, cartilage, etc.) as well as on the laser being used.

Visible spectrum laser (argon and KTP) energy absorption by tissue is partially dependent on tissue color. For example, for soft tissue work, chromophores of hemoglobin and melanin absorb most of the energy. Tissues having a lighter color will reflect most of the energy from the laser. Energy absorption from the invisible carbon dioxide laser is primarily by intracellular and extracellular water, which is instantly converted to steam.

The magnitude of the laser tissue interaction can be regulated by the laser's power output, the power density, and the energy fluence. Power can be defined as the time rate at which energy is emitted and is expressed in watts. The power output is directly adjusted by the control panel on the laser console.

Laser energy is delivered through a focusing lens. Power density is a measure of the intensity or concentration of the laser beam spot size. Power density can be expressed as the ratio of power to the surface area of the spot size and is expressed in terms of watts per square centimeter:

Power density = power (watts) / area of spot size (cm²)

Area of spot size is $\pi r^2$, where $r$ equals the spot size radius in centimeters. Thus, it can be seen that power density is inversely proportional to the square of the radius of the spot size. For any specific power output, changes in the spot size can have a tremendous effect on power density.

Fluence can be expressed with the formula

Fluence (joules) = power (watts) × exposure time (seconds) / area of spot size (cm²)

As the fluence increases, so does the volume of affected tissue. The thermal energy having an impact on tissue rises dramatically as the time of exposure increases.

There are four factors that determine laser–tissue interactions:

1. The laser wavelength (frequency)

2. The absorption characteristics of the tissue

3. The temporal parameters of the laser energy delivered

4. The mechanism of the laser delivery

An incident beam of laser radiation on tissue can have one of the following effects:

1. Reflection

2. Absorption

3. Scattering

4. Transmission

The ideal qualities of a laser for use during a stapedectomy are the following:

1. Precise optics are required to focus the laser beam at the place required.

2. The laser should be able to vaporize either the bone or the collagen at the oval window in a predictable manner.

3. The thermal footprint of the laser should not be beyond (deeper than) the site of application. If it did penetrate beyond the site of application, it would cause thermal damage to the utricle and the saccule beneath.

4. The laser should not heat the perilymph.

## OPTICAL PROPERTIES

### Visible Lasers

The short wavelength lasers (argon = 488 or 514 nm; KTP = 532 nm) have ideal optical properties for microscopic surgery. The KTP laser is produced by passing an Nd:YAG laser output through a KTP crystal, which doubles the frequency (halves the wavelength) of the laser light. The KTP laser is generally a Q switched laser. The argon laser is produced by excitation of argon gas, yielding two possible laser bands at 488 nm (blue light) and 514 nm (green light). The light can be delivered from the laser source to the microscope-mounted micromanipulator through an optical fiber and can be focused to a spot size of 0.5 mm or smaller. The light of the aiming beam and the light of the working beam are the same spot size, and their point of impact is identical; that is to say, they are parfocal and coaxial. Initially, Perkins (1980) and McGee (1983) used microscope-mounted lasers. In 1990, Gherini and Horn introduced a handheld Endo-Otoprobe (HGM Medical Lasers Systems, Salt Lake City, UT) to deliver an argon laser beam; this provided further refinement to the convenient use of lasers in stapedectomy.

### Infrared Lasers

Currently, long-wavelength carbon dioxide ($CO_2$) laser light (10,600 nm) can only be transmitted to the microscope via a series of carefully aligned mirrors and lenses. The infrared $CO_2$ laser is invisible to the naked eye, so a visible laser aiming beam is needed. For this purpose, a helium-neon laser is used. The $CO_2$ laser is delivered in a CW mode and can also be used in a superpulsed mode (a chopped variation of CW) to produce higher peak energies but less thermal dissipation in tissue.

## ADVANTAGES OF THE $CO_2$ LASER

The $CO_2$ laser has near ideal tissue absorption characteristics because the laser energy is absorbed by water. The water component of bone, for example, is approximately 60%. At the high-power density setting, the pulsed laser vaporizes bone and releases heat and tissue into the vapor plume. Because the $CO_2$ laser energy is absorbed by water, it does not penetrate.

## DISADVANTAGES OF THE $CO_2$ LASER

Disadvantages of the $CO_2$ laser include the following:

1. The laser apparatus is cumbersome.

2. Increased working distance exists between the microscope and the operative site.

3. Diminished light through the microscope is common because of the use of the beam splitter.

4. The aiming beam and the working beam do not have the same wavelength, so it becomes difficult to focus both together at the same spot.

In short, the $CO_2$ laser can be said to have optimal tissue characteristics but suboptimal optical characteristics for use in stapedectomy (Poe 2000).

## ADVANTAGES OF VISIBLE LASERS

The advantages of visible lasers include the convenience of the handheld probe and the fact that the spot size can be chosen accurately.

## DISADVANTAGES OF VISIBLE LASERS

Visible light lasers depend on char formation to begin creation of a rosette (fenestra) on the footplate. The char absorbs laser energy and creates heat. The laser energy can pass through (either directly or by scatter) and injure the neural tissue of the utricle or saccule.

## WHICH LASER SHOULD BE USED FOR STAPEDECTOMY?

Presently, there is no ideal laser. The visible lasers, especially the argon Endo-Otoprobe, have excellent optical precision, superior to the $CO_2$ laser. The $CO_2$ laser, however, has superior interaction of laser energy with bone, collagen, and perilymph (Fig. 9–1). Fluency threshold studies confirm that 15 to 20 times more argon or KTP energy is required to ablate bone (Lesinski and Newrock 1993). Transmission spectroscopy studies of both collagen and bone further verified the selective absorption of infrared electromagnetic energy compared with visible light (DiBartolomeo 1981). Finally, ther-

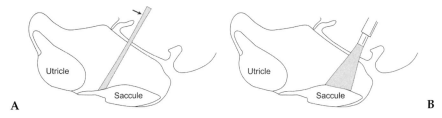

**Figure 9–1** **(A)** Schematic representation showing how the laser beam from the micromanipulator has the potential risk of damaging structures proximal and distal to the target because the rate of power density falloff on either side is small. **(B)** The Endo-Otoprobe has a larger angle of divergence and a rapid power density falloff, thus reducing the risk of damage to structures both proximal and distal. (From Friedman MD. Surgical management of otosclerosis: Primary stapedectomy surgery. *Operative Techniques in Otolaryngology—Head and Neck Surgery.* 1998;9(1):55. Used with permission.)

mocouple experiments show that, should correct energy parameters and surgical care during surgery be taken, both visible and invisible (infrared) lasers can be used safely for stapedectomy (Perkins 1980).

A pulsed $CO_2$ laser beam is ideal for revision stapedectomy because infrared lasers are well absorbed by collagen. Because visible lasers are poorly absorbed by collagen and pass readily through perilymph, they are less preferable for revision stapedectomy.

## IDEAL SITUATIONS FOR LASER STAPEDECTOMY

Situations that are ideal for laser stapedectomy include
    Revision stapedectomy (Fig. 9–2)
    Obliterative footplate
    Primary stapedectomy is also an ideal situation because in stapedectomy the first surgery is the best chance for an optimal outcome.

## ADVANTAGES OF LASER STAPEDECTOMY

The advantages of laser stapedectomy include the following:

1. A precise fenestra can be created in the oval window.

2. Laser stapedectomy avoids trauma to the inner ear. The incidences of vertigo, sensorineural hearing loss, and tinnitus are much less likely.

3. A floating footplate is more likely to occur with manual stapedectomy where the surgeon attempts to create a fenestra without the use of a laser. The use of a laser lowers the chance of a floating footplate occurring.

4. Laser stapedectomy results in good hemostasis.

5. Good long-term results in terms of hearing can be expected following laser stapedectomy.

Wiet et al (1997) have shown a statistically significant benefit by using the laser for primary and revision stapedectomies. Other authors (De la

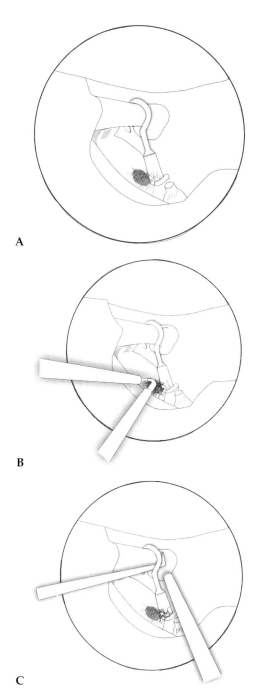

**A**

**B**

**C**

**Figure 9–2** **(A)** Depiction of a prosthesis that has migrated and has adhesions. **(B)** Diagram of the Endo-Otoprobe vaporizing the adhesions. A suction aspirator removes the laser plumes while adhesiolysis is carried out. **(C)** Once adhesiolysis is carried out, the prosthesis can be safely removed. *(From Friedman MD. Surgical management of otosclerosis: Revision stapedectomy surgery.* Operative Techniques in Otolaryngology—Head and Neck Surgery. *1998; 9(2):89. Used with permission.)*

Cruz and Fayyad 2000; Nissen 1998; Silverstein et al 1994) have also reported on the use of laser in stapedectomy; in these reports, the authors have suggested that the laser made stapedectomy less difficult technically, which in turn led to better results.

## COMPARISON OF LASERS

The visible wavelength lasers (argon and KTP 532) have the practical advantage of precision because the aiming beam and the working beam are one and the same (Table 9–1). The aiming beam is clear and crisp and allows precision. The $CO_2$ laser is invisible; therefore, a separate visible-light aiming beam (helium-neon) is needed. This aiming beam is coaxial and focuses in a different plane from the $CO_2$ laser because of the difference in wavelength; this has the potential to cause misalignment, with a resulting greater margin of error. This necessitates that the $CO_2$ laser and its helium-neon aiming beam be calibrated precisely and frequently to ensure accuracy.

Argon and KTP lasers are color-dependent for tissue absorption; for these lasers, peak absorption is dark red. For tissues that are not red, such as bone and cartilage, a significant amount of laser energy is reflected rather than absorbed. This is usually overcome by placing minute quantities of blood in the field or applying several well-spaced bursts to get a darker char to increase energy absorption. This problem does not occur with the $CO_2$ laser because absorption by water and tissue is not color dependent.

The visible wavelength lasers have two modes of delivery: a micromanipulator attached to the microscope and a handheld probe. The handheld probe allows a greater angle of divergence of the laser beam, which allows for rapid deterioration of power density and therefore must be placed very close to the tissue that is to be operated upon. Because it must be placed directly in the operating field, it can on occasion obstruct visibility. In the case of the micromanipulator, the angle of the laser beam is less divergent and does not obstruct vision.

The $CO_2$ laser cannot be delivered through fiberoptics; it is delivered instead through a micromanipulator system. The micromanipulator system has recently been made less cumbersome and allows the optical chamber to be attached to the side of the microscope.

**Table 9–1  Comparison of Lasers**

|  | **Argon** | **KTP 532** | **$CO_2$** |
|---|---|---|---|
| Medium | gas | crystal | gas |
| Wavelength | 488–514 nm | 532 nm | 10,600 nm |
| Color | blue-green | green | invisible (infrared) |
| Smallest spot size | 0.150 mm | 0.150 mm | 0.150 mm |
| Delivery | handheld probe or micromanipulator | handheld probe or micromanipulator | micromanipulator |
| Absorption | pigment | pigment | water |

## BEAM VERSUS PROBE

With the beam directed from the microscope, it is possible to see exactly where the fenestra will be placed. With a handheld probe, however, vision may be obstructed by the probe itself. Furthermore, unless the probe itself is touching the footplate, the size of the fenestra tends to vary, and the completeness of the vaporization tends to become erratic because of the varying spot size. With contact vaporization, however, there is the risk of the laser physically penetrating the thin footplate. In this respect, the KTP laser microbeam device mounted on the microscope results in extremely accurate spot placement and uniformity in the fenestra created on the footplate.

## VESTIBULAR SAFETY

Lasers, in both the invisible and the visible spectrum, appear to be reasonably safe for use during stapedectomy. Disturbances due to the thermal effects of the laser were initially greatly feared, but most reports have found lasers safe and effective. The lack of significant thermal effects seems to result from several factors. It is likely that most of the heat is dissipated in the vaporization of bone of the footplate, and is further reduced by the suction tip. Additionally, the laser energy is delivered in a series of pulses with intervals of rest in between, thus preventing heat buildup. Furthermore, the laser beam is in focus on the lateral side of the footplate, and it immediately defocuses beyond the focal point. Calculations (Perkins 1994) suggest that the energy density of the defocused beam decreases significantly by the time it arrives at the saccule, which is approximately 1.8 mm away from the footplate. Nonetheless, the surgeon should avoid firing the laser beam into the open vestibule, especially if blood has entered it, because blood could have the potential to absorb the laser energy and thus cause thermal damage to the saccule.

## SAFETY OF THE FACIAL NERVE

Many surgeons have voiced concern over the safety of the facial nerve during laser use. When the recommended parameters of the laser pulse are adhered to, however, a single pulse is unlikely to penetrate the bone of the fallopian canal. The bone of the fallopian canal is much thicker than the footplate, and the white neural sheath is less likely to absorb the heat from the laser. Of course, due care should be taken at all times to avoid exposing the facial nerve to the laser beam. Special care should be taken if the facial nerve is dehiscent or bifid.

## SURGICAL TECHNIQUE

$CO_2$ laser stapedotomy is usually performed under local anesthesia with intravenous sedation. The steps to expose the stapes are the same for standard stapedectomy:

1. The tympanic flap is elevated in the usual way.
2. The posterior canal wall is curetted away until the entire stapes is fully exposed.

3. The chorda tympani is preserved.

4. The malleus, incus, and stapes are inspected, and their mobility is tested. The middle ear is inspected and examined for other abnormalities.

5. The distance between the undersurface of the incus and the stapes footplate is measured.

6. The prosthesis length should be 0.25 mm longer.

7. The stapedius tendon and the posterior crus are vaporized.

8. The anterior crus is fractured.

9. The incudostapedial joint is separated by a right-angled pick, the stapes is fractured, and the superstructure is removed.

10. Energy parameters for the Unilase $CO_2$ laser are as follows: spot size 0.3 mm, power 2.0 watts, mode: Superpulse, pulse duration 0.1 second; or spot size 0.6 mm, power 4.0 watts, mode: Superpulse, pulse duration 0.2 second.

11. A 0.6 mm opening is created in the posterior part of the footplate (a footplate of normal thickness normally requires two hits to create a fenestra of the desired size).

12. The prosthesis is inserted.

13. The prosthesis should extend 0.2 mm below the footplate.

14. A seal is placed over the fenestra around the piston.

15. The patient's hearing is checked intraoperatively. The patient is asked if he or she experiences vertigo, tinnitus, or any other such complaint.

16. The tympanomeatal flap is replaced, and the external auditory canal is packed.

## Results: Virgin (Primary) Surgery

### Conductive Hearing Loss

Almost all authors conclude that with whatever laser they use, hearing results are uniformly good and are superior to those performed through conventional techniques without the use of laser (Lesinski and Stein 1989; Perkins 1980).

Lesinski and Newrock (1993) reported on 100 consecutive patients who had undergone $CO_2$ laser stapedectomy. They were examined 1 to 3 years postoperatively. In this series, 91% of patients maintained an air-bone gap within 10 dB or better, 95% within 15 dB. Three patients had an air-bone gap of 20 dB.

### Sensorineural Hearing Loss

No patient in the Lesinski and Newrock (1993) series was found to have a sensorineural hearing loss in the speech range of 500, 1000, 2000, or 3000 Hz. McGee et al (1993) reported on 185 KTP laser revision stapedotomy cases, of which 77 involved actual removal of an existing prosthesis. The surgery also involved the creation of a fresh, new fenestra and the placement of a prosthesis. Of these 77 cases, 80.5% had an air-bone gap closure to within 10 dB, and 92.3% had an air-bone gap closure to within 20 dB. There were no dead ears, and no patients reported an increase in their tinnitus postoperatively.

## COMPLICATIONS

### Perilymph Fistula

No patients in the Lesinski and Newrock (1993) series went on to develop a perilymphatic fistula.

### Vestibular Symptoms

Intraoperatively, no patient developed dizziness. Within 4 hours, 13 developed mild dizziness. All symptoms resolved, however, within 1 month of surgery.

## REVISION STAPEDECTOMY SURGERY WITH LASER

Lesinski and Newrock (1993) reported better hearing results in those who were found to have a normal malleus and incus at the time of revision surgery. Ninety percent of patients maintained an air-bone gap to within 10 dB. For those patients who presented with incus erosion or malleus fixation, the results were poorer. No patient developed a worse speech reception threshold. No patient developed a significant sensorineural hearing loss.

## NEWER LASERS FOR THE USE OF STAPEDECTOMY

The search for an ideal otological laser has been directed toward development of a laser with good water absorption characteristics that could be delivered through a fiberoptic cable. The search has focused on alternative wavelengths for lasers in the midinfrared range where water absorption is good.

### Pulsed Infrared Lasers

To date, the emerging lasers in the midinfrared region have been pulsed lasers. Pulsed lasers work by storing a large amount of energy that is suddenly dissipated in a massive release that generates the laser emission in very short bursts. These high-energy bursts rapidly exceed tissue vaporization levels with efficient tissue ablation that reduces the total energy required for ablation compared with continuous wave lasers. Pulsed lasers lose less energy to adjacent thermal spread, yielding a better quality perforation of the oval window. The high-energy bursts over a brief period of time produce a transient plasma explosion with nonlinear (out of proportion for the amount of energy) acoustic effects not found in CW lasers that follow only linear photothermal properties. Pulsed lasers have highly desirable wavelengths and are excellent at bone cutting. The acoustic shock wave, however, has been found to be a potential serious barrier for their use within the ear.

Esenaliev et al (1993) found that the shorter the pulse, the greater the acoustic effect, particularly when the duration of the pulse was less than the duration of the stress relaxation time as the tissue recoiled from each pressure wave. The pulsed or explosive ejection of tissue ablation products caused a compression and rarefaction recoil pulse that, propagated through tissues, could cause significant injury even at remote distances from the site of ablation. All of the acoustic effects caused tissue stresses and generated energy below levels required for tissue ablation, so no secondary vaporization would be expected, but widespread necrosis could result.

## Erbium Laser

The erbium (Er) laser is available in two types of pulsed (< 1 μm) lasers that are very similar. Er:YAG has a wavelength of 2.94 μm, and Er:YSGG (yttrium-scandium-gallium-garnet) has a wavelength of 2.79 μm. Erbium has high-fluence pulses from its short duration and makes very sharp vaporization craters with little adjacent thermal necrosis.

The erbium laser is currently being investigated because of its clean bone-cutting characteristics and because it has a wavelength of 2.9 μm, close to the maximal peak of water absorption (3.00 μm) in the infrared spectrum. Shah et al (1996) examined the erbium laser and found that 10 pulses of the laser on the footplate produced a 2.0° elevation in temperature. It was noted that the erbium laser was capable of precise bony ablation and very limited collateral damage, with much less char than either CW or superpulsed $CO_2$ lasers. The erbium laser was intensely absorbed by water and collagen and also by bone minerals such as calcium phosphate and hydroxyapatite. The excellent absorption of the laser energy meant that the majority of the energy was consumed by tissue ablation and ejection of debris, leaving minimal residual energy to dissipate into adjacent tissues. Hemostasis was limited. The erbium laser worked best on very small vessels. It was also noted that a loud popping sound occurred when the laser impacted the bone. This was indicative of a significant shock wave phenomenon.

Jovanovic et al (1995) found that the Er:YSGG laser produced a 3.6° celsius elevation in temperature from the footplate, and the $CO_2$ laser produced an 8.8° celsius temperature increase. The researchers were concerned that the shock waves could be introduced into the perilymph with the potential to damage the inner ear structures. They also found that the Er:YSGG laser created well-formed fenestra in the oval window. The Er:YSGG laser requires two to four times less total energy than the $CO_2$ laser.

Nagel (1997) used the Er:YAG laser in stapedectomy, of which 32 were small fenestra surgeries. His data showed that 8 of 32 patients had a hearing loss greater than 10 dB at 4000 or 8000 Hz, which meets the American Academy of Otolaryngology—Head and Neck Surgery (1995) criteria for hearing loss reporting. However, Huber et al (2001) and Kecke et al (2002) reported their findings on patients who had undergone stapedectomy using the Er:YAG laser and found no risk to the inner ear.

## Thulium Laser

Bottrill et al (1994) published their findings of a pulsed thulium (Tm:YAG 2.01 μm) laser. It was a flashlamp pumped, solid-state laser using a chromium-sensitized Cr:YAG crystal doped with thulium ions and delivered through a quartz fiber. The Tm:YAG laser had many similarities to the erbium laser but was less precise in cutting bone. It produced an audible acoustic shock that was significant. On human cadaveric bone, it was found that dry bone could actually ignite. Further work was not pursued because of the acoustic shock and the potential for flame.

## Diode Lasers

New semiconductor diode lasers, which are fiber delivered, inexpensive, and available in CW or pulsed modes, are available in recent times. The clinically available wavelengths, however, between 800 and 1000 nm fall between hemoglobin and water absorption peaks. Although they are useful for pigmented bodies, they cause deep extensive thermal damage.

## LASER-ASSISTED ENDOSCOPIC STAPEDIOPLASTY

This technique was described by Poe (2000), who performed 11 laser-assisted endoscopic stapedioplasty without prosthesis. Poe used a prototype argon laser endoscope (Endo Optiks) that had been especially designed to his specifications. The endoscopes used were Hopkins rod 1.9 mm 0 and 30 degree wide-angle endoscopes (Karl Storz, Culver City, CA); the 10K pixel 0.9 mm optical density (OD) fiberoptic endoscope (Endo Optiks, Little Silver, NJ); and the gradient index (GRIN) (0.5 mm lens in an overall package of 1.2 mm OD) endoscopes. Images were presented on a Sony Trinitron 13 inch color video monitor. The Hopkins rod endoscopes were fitted with a telecam video camera head and Dx cam processor (Karl Storz). The fiberoptic scope used an internal camera in the laser endoscopic unit (Endo Optiks). The GRIN lens was fitted with a video camera using an Elmo processor (Elmo Corporation, Tokyo, Japan).

The endoscope was fitted with a 200 µm diameter argon laser fiber protruding from the endoscope's distal tip for a distance of 3 mm. The laser fiber was coupled to the argon laser (HGM, Salt Lake City, UT). Fog Away antifog solution (Technol Medical Products Inc., Fort Worth, TX) was applied to the endoscope tip. The tympanic flap is elevated in the conventional way with the aid of the microscope. The middle ear is entered, and the microscope is then removed from the operating field.

Next, the laser endoscope is introduced into the field, and the field is viewed from the monitor. If the otosclerotic focus involves only the anterior half of the footplate, then laser-assisted stapedioplasty is thought to be feasible.

The anterior crus is then lysed with the laser, with the laser power settings at 2.0 W and 0.2 second, using the laser in near-contact with the bone. Division of the crus is confirmed. The laser setting is then used to make a row of burns on the footplate to separate it at the junction between the anterior and middle thirds. Once the footplate division is complete, the posterior crus is palpated to ensure that the footplate is mobile. Once it has been confirmed that the footplate is now mobile, the footplate is covered with perichondrium, the tympanic flap is repositioned, and the surgery is terminated.

## GRADIENT INDEX ENDOSCOPES

Gradient index (GRIN) has provided a means for developing ever smaller diameter rigid lens endoscopes The GRIN lenses have an axially or radially variable index of refraction that permits small diameter construction. However, they suffered from distortions such as spherical and chromatic aberrations, which were thought to be due to the low number of optical elements It was only in 1984 that diffusion components in the Selfoc device were improved sufficiently to construct useful rigid scopes in diameters less than 2 mm. GRIN endoscopes use radially variable index of refraction components. The Hopkins rod lens system uses multiple lens elements fixed in a rigid housing and operate largely on ray optics. GRIN endoscopes are governed by both ray and wave optics and are fundamentally constructed of only two elements. They are an objective lens and a much longer relay lens. The two are cemented to each other end to end to eliminate any air interface between them. The walls of the relay lens create a natural aperture stop, and the lengths of the two lenses are designed so that the objective lens is one quarter period of the relay lens. The relay lens must be of any length that is an integral number of half periods.

## Advantages/Disadvantages

The advantages of GRIN endoscopes include their small size, brightness, and economical costs. Disadvantages include their reduced field of view, vignetting, (small portion of the big picture) and reduced resolution.

## LASER STAPEDOTOMY MINUS PROSTHESIS: ABSENCE OF REFIXATION

Silverstein et al (2002) attempted to determine the percentage of patients with otosclerosis who could successfully undergo a laser stapedotomy minus prosthesis (LSTAMP) over a 5 year period. In essence, this is the same procedure as described by Poe (2000). The authors also attempted to determine the percentage of patients in whom refixation reoccurs. Theirs was a retrospective study involving 136 patients (137 ears). For the laser stapedotomy, a handheld probe was used to vaporize the anterior crus and perform a linear stapedotomy across the anterior one third of the footplate. If otosclerosis was confined to the fissula ante fenestram, the stapes became completely mobile. Thus, only the posterior crus was now connected with the newly mobilized posterior portion of the footplate. The stapedectomy opening was sealed with adipose tissue. Pure tone audiometry, with appropriate masking and auditory discrimination testing, was performed before surgery, 6 weeks after surgery, and every year thereafter. Of the 137 ears, favorable anatomy and minimal otosclerosis allowed 46 (33.6%) to undergo LSTAMP. Fifty-seven ears (41.6%) could not undergo the procedure because of extensive otosclerosis. The remaining 34 ears (24.8%) did not receive LSTAMP because of anatomic or technical difficulties. Of the 34 LSTAMP group with more than 4 months' follow-up, the average air-bone gap was closed from a mean of 22 dB to 6 dB 6 weeks postoperatively. Follow-up ranged from 5 months to 53 months (mean 767 days; DSD 437 days). The long-term air-bone gap improved slightly to an average of 5 dB (SD 6 dB) in comparison with the sixth postoperative week value. Silverstein et al concluded that LSTAMP, a minimally invasive procedure, has a very low incidence of refixation, as evidenced by a lack of the reappearance of a conductive hearing loss. The success of this procedure depends on the correct selection of patients. The authors performed the procedure upon 33.6% of patients who underwent primary stapes surgery. LSTAMP seems to offer a viable alternative to conventional stapedectomy and offers good results without refixation of the footplate over an extended period of time.

## SUMMARY

$CO_2$ laser energy (10.6 μm) is nearly completely absorbed by collagen and bone. The $CO_2$ laser has certain disadvantages, such as cumbersome delivery apparatus, increased working distance, and diminished light because of the use of the beam splitter. The aiming beam and the laser beam have to be calibrated frequently to ensure accuracy. However, the $CO_2$ laser is the ideal tool to use in revision stapedectomy surgery.

Visible lasers such as argon and KTP are poorly absorbed by tissues that are not colored red. This can be overcome by placing minute amounts of blood on the site to be addressed by the laser. Multiple laser pulses will create a char that will absorb the laser energy. More importantly, they can be delivered through a convenient handheld probe. Visible lasers are ideal for primary stapes surgery. Newer lasers such as erbium are being developed to overcome the disadvantages of older lasers.

Many authors, using different lasers, have all reported excellent results. They have all reported a good safety profile with the lasers used. Laser stapedectomy has, to a certain extent, reduced technical difficulties of a very technical surgery. It must be said, however, that the laser, whichever one is used, is only as good as the hand that wields it.

## REFERENCES

Bottrill I, Perrault DF, Pankratov MM, Poe DS. Thulium:YAG laser for stapes surgery: Preliminary observations. *SPIE Int Soc England.* 1994;2128:23–30.

De la Cruz A, Fayyad JN. Revision stapedectomy. *Otolaryngol Head Neck Surg.* 2000;123:728–732.

DiBartolomeo J. Argon and $CO_2$ lasers in otolaryngology: Which one, when and why? *Laryngoscope.* 1981;91(suppl 26):1–16.

DiBartolomeo JR, Ellis M. The argon laser in otology. *Laryngoscope.* 1980;90: 1786–1796.

Esenaliev RO, Oraevsky AA, Letokhov VS, Karabutov AA, Malinsky TV. Studies of acoustical and shock waves in the pulsed laser ablation of biotissue. *Lasers Surg Med.* 1993;13:470–484.

Gherini S, Horn KL. Small fenestra laser stapedectomy utilizing a handheld argon laser in obliterative otosclerosis. Paper presented at the Western Section, The Triologic Society, January 6, 1990; Pebble Beach, CA.

Huber A, Linder T, Fisch U. Is the Er:YAG laser damaging to inner ear function? *Otol Neurotol.* 2001;22:311–315.

Jovanovic S, Schonfeld U, Prapavat V, et al. Effects of pulsed laser systems on stapes footplate. *Lasers Surg Med.* 1995;21:341–350.

Kecke T, Wiebe M, Rettinger G, Riechelmann H. Safety of the erbium:yttrium aluminium-garnet laser in stapes surgery in otosclerosis. *Otol Neurotol.* 2002;23:21–24.

Lesinski SG, Newrock R. Carbon dioxide lasers for otosclerosis. *Otolaryngol Clin N Am.* 1993;26:417–441.

Lesinski SG, Stein J. $CO_2$ laser stapedotomy. *Laryngoscope.* 1989; 99(suppl 46):20–23.

McGee T. The argon laser in surgery for chronic ear disease and otosclerosis. *Laryngoscope.* 1983;93:1177–1182.

McGee TM. Lasers in otology. *Otolaryngol Clin N Am.* 1989;22:233–238.

McGee TM, Diat Ordaz EA, Kartush JM. The role of KTP laser in revision stapedotomy. *Otolaryngol Head Neck Surg.* 1993;109:839–843.

Nagel D. The Er:YAG laser in ear surgery: First clinical results. *Lasers Surg Med.* 1997;21:79–87.

Nissen RL. Argon laser in difficult stapedotomy cases. *Laryngoscope.* 1998;108: 1669–1673.

Perkins R. Laser stapedotomy for otosclerosis. *Laryngoscope.* 1980;90:228–241.

Perkins R. Laser stapedotomy. In: Brackmann D, Shelton C, Arriaga MA, eds. *Otologic Surgery.* Philadelphia: WB Saunders; 1994:313–329.

Poe DS. Laser assisted endoscopic stapedectomy: A prospective study. *Laryngoscope.* 2000;110(suppl 95):1–37.

Sataloff J. Experimental use of the laser in otosclerotic stapes. *Arch Otolaryngol, Head Neck Surg.* 1967;85:58–60.

Shah UK, Poe DS, Rebeiz EE, Perrault DF, et al. Erbium laser in middle ear surgery: In vivo and in vitro animal study. *Laryngoscope.* 1996;106:418–422.

Silverstein H, Bendet E, Rosenberg S, Nichols M. Revision stapes surgery with and without laser: A comparison. *Laryngoscope.* 1994;104:1431–1438.

Silverstein H, Jackson LE, Conlon WS, Rosenberg SI, Thompson JH. Laser stapedotomy minus prosthesis (Laser STAMP): Absence of refixation. *Otol Neurotol.* 2002;23(2):152–157.

Smith MFW, McElveen JE. *Neurological Surgery of the Ear.* St. Louis: Mosby Yearbook; 1992:131–162.

Stahle J, Hoeberg L, Engstrom B. The laser as a tool in inner ear surgery. *Acta Otolaryngol.* 1972;73:27–37.

Wiet RJ, Kubek DC, Lemberg P, Byskosh A. A meta-analysis review of revision surgery with argon laser: Effectiveness and safety. *Am J Otol.* 1997;18:166–171.

# Chapter *10*

# Stapedectomy

Stapedectomy is indicated when the patient is suspected of having otosclerosis with a bone conduction level of 0 to 25 dB in the speech range and an air conduction loss of 45 to 65 dB. The air-bone gap should be at least 15 dB. If the air-bone gap is less than 20 dB, the disease may be early and actively growing, and the patient's hearing may not be significantly impaired.

## FAR ADVANCED OTOSCLEROSIS

Patients with hearing losses in the 90 to 100 dB range may be suitable for stapedectomy because this surgery may enable them to use a hearing aid. Far advanced otosclerosis (FAO) is defined as no measurable air or bone conduction, or air conduction no better than 95 dB and bone conduction at 55 to 60 dB at one frequency only (Lippy 1994). In a retrospective study, Shea et al (1999) described their results with stapedectomy in 78 ears with FAO. Their follow-up ranged over a period from 1 to 21 years, with a mean follow-up of 5 years. All patients had air conduction (AC) and bone conduction (BC) tested. Rinne's test was performed with a 256 Hz magnesium tuning fork. The pure tone average for AC and BC was computed for 500, 1000, and 2000 Hz. Hearing improvement was defined as air-bone gap closure to 10 dB or less and/or AC improvement of 20 dB or more, with no decline in speech discrimination scores greater than 10%. In their results, Shea et al reported that hearing improvement was achieved in 52 of 78 ears (66.7%). In group 1, AC was greater than 90 dB, BC was greater than 60 dB, and hearing improved in 26 of 32 ears (81.2%).

In group 2, AC was greater than 90 dB, and no measurable BC and hearing improved in 11 of 16 ears (68.8%). In group 3, there was no measurable AC and BC greater than 60 dB, and hearing improved in two of four ears (50%). In group 4, there was no measurable AC and BC, and hearing improved in 11 of 26 ears (42.3%). Nonmeasurable BC became measurable in 42.9% of ears, nonmeasurable AC became measurable in 73.3% of ears, and all of these became aidable after surgery. The authors concluded that a negative Rinne's test result with a 256 Hz magnesium tuning fork proved to be the best test to separate FAO sensorineural hearing loss of other causes. Stapedectomy benefited most of their patients with profound hearing loss caused by FAO, especially in those ears with some measurable hearing by air conduction.

Lippy et al (1998) examined word recognition scores (WRSs) following stapedectomy for FAO. The WRS changes were examined to determine whether they were consistent with acclimatization or recovery from auditory deprivation changes that have been seen after the restoration of sound by amplification. A total of 24 patients who were suffering from FAO were analyzed retrospectively. One month following surgery, the mean WRS had improved 16.5%. The WRS continued to improve an additional 12% or more for 17 of 24 patients (71%) within 2 years after their initial postoperative hearing test. The mean WRS improvement within 2 years of the initial postoperative test was 16.2%. The authors arrived at the conclusion that initial WRS changes were attributed to hearing thresholds no longer remaining at or staying beyond audiometric limits. Additional WRS changes were consistent with reports of acclimatization or recovery from audiometric deprivation that have been seen after hearing aid use.

In their series of patients with FAO, Khalifa et al (1998) also concluded that cochlear implantation is not the best treatment for all profoundly deaf patients because some are better off with stapedectomy.

## STAPEDECTOMY IN CHILDREN

Initially, stapedectomy was thought to be an unsuitable procedure to be performed on children. Its effectiveness in children previously received less scrutiny in the literature. However, there has been a gathering body of evidence that includes children as candidates for stapedectomy (House et al 1980; Namyslowski et al 2001; Szymanski et al 2001).

De la Cruz et al (1999) reported on 95 ears of 81 patients younger than 18 years of age who had undergone stapedectomy from 1980 to 1994. There were 83 primary stapedectomies and 12 revision stapedectomies. Two groups were identified: congenital stapedial fixation and juvenile otosclerosis. Patients with congenital stapes fixation had an earlier onset of hearing loss (3 vs 10 ears, $p < .001$), a greater incidence of abnormalities of the malleus and incus (25% vs 3%, $p < .001$), and a slighter greater preoperative air-bone gap (35.2 ± 12.9 vs 27.8 ± 8.9, $p < .001$). Overall, 79% of primary cases and 89% of revision cases had an improvement in hearing, with mean postoperative air-bone gaps of 15 and 22 dB, respectively. The gap did not widen significantly during the entire length of follow-up (mean 72 months). In primary cases, 59.1% obtained a postoperative air-bone gap of 10 dB or less. Eighty-two percent of children operated on for otosclerosis obtained excellent results (postoperative air-bone gap $\leq$ 10 dB), compared with only 44% of children with congenital stapedial fixation ($p = .02$). In revision surgery, 29% of children obtained excellent results. Poorer results in both cases of congenital stapedial fixation and revision stapedectomy appear to be related to the greater incidence of associated anomalies of the malleus and incus.

In their study on stapedectomy that was performed on 47 children, Lippy et al (1998) confirmed that stapedectomy can be safely performed on children. Murphy and Wallis (1996) compared the results of stapedectomy in pediatric patients for otosclerosis and tympanosclerosis. They reviewed retrospectively 14 patients (15 ears) who underwent stapedectomy at their institute from

1993 to 1995. In five ears, stapedectomy was performed for tympanosclerosis; nine patients had otosclerosis, and one had Treacher Collins syndrome. Children with otosclerosis who underwent stapedectomy had an average postoperative air-bone gap of 16 dB, with an average air conduction hearing improvement of 17.6 dB. Children with tympanosclerosis who underwent stapedectomy had an average air-bone gap of 14 dB, with an average air conduction hearing improvement of 28 dB. The authors concluded that stapedectomy was a safe and effective treatment for children suffering from otosclerosis and tympanosclerosis.

Millman et al (1996) acknowledged that although good results of stapedectomy in children are rewarding in themselves, the possible complications that may occur are devastating. In their study, 31 patients 21 years of age or younger underwent stapedectomy at their institute. The average age at surgery was 16 years. Millman et al collected clinical and audiological data over a mean follow-up period of 25 years. They reported that there was no statistically significant difference in the air-bone gap when comparing the immediate postoperative gap (measured 2 months after stapedectomy) with the last recorded (mean 25 years after stapedectomy) audiogram. Fifty percent of the ears operated on maintained an air-bone gap within 10 dB at the last follow-up, and an additional 40% maintained a 10 to 20 dB gap. The authors concluded that stapedectomy was an effective method for closing the air-bone gap in children and that the long-term results equal those that can be achieved in adults. Their review represents the largest population with the longest follow-up in children who underwent stapedectomy for otosclerosis.

The main fear of stapedectomy in children was that their sport and athletic activities would be limited following this procedure. In other words, it was feared that the normal rough and tumble of childhood, middle ear infections, and middle ear effusions would adversely affect the results of stapedectomy. These studies show, however, that if children keep to reasonable activity without major head trauma, then stapedectomy is a safe and effective procedure. Of course, it is well to caution the children and their caregivers away from certain sports like boxing, football, and wrestling, where head trauma is an inherent risk. All respiratory tract infections need to be treated promptly, especially in those children who have undergone stapedectomy.

## STAPEDECTOMY IN THE ELDERLY

The role of stapedectomy in the elderly has been debated. Arguments against stapedectomy have cited an increased risk of sensorineural hearing loss and vestibular problems, inferring that an aging cochlea is more susceptible to surgical trauma (Awengen 1993). Other studies (Mann et al 1996; Vartiainen 1995) refuted these arguments with findings that demonstrate that both hearing results and complication rates show no significant difference between the elderly and younger age groups.

Lippy and colleagues (Lippy et al 1996) reviewed the effectiveness of stapedectomy in those patients who were 70 years and older. A total of 154 patients were studied, including 11 patients with profound hearing loss with long-standing otosclerosis. Ages of the patients ranged from 70 to 92 years. Lippy et al reported that stapedectomy in the elderly gave a 90.9% success rate, which they found was comparable to the rate for a younger age group of patients who had undergone stapedectomy. Albera et al (2001) also concluded that stapedectomy was a safe and rewarding procedure that can be effectively performed in the elderly. Stapedectomy serves not only to reduce a handicap but also to improve the quality of life in the elderly. Furthermore, those who are profoundly deaf can benefit from amplification following stapedectomy.

Given the success of primary stapedectomy, what then is the role of revision stapedectomy in the elderly? This was the question that Lippy et al (2002) attempted to answer in their study. They compared 123 elderly patients with a randomly selected group of 120 younger patients. Both groups had undergone revision stapedectomy by the same surgeon. The authors reported that the success rate was 70.8% for the elderly group and 67.6% for the younger group. Surgical findings were generally the same for both groups. Lippy et al thus concluded that advanced age should not be a contraindication to revision stapedectomy.

## STAPEDECTOMY IN COMBAT PILOTS AND IN DIVERS

Katzav et al (1996) reported on nine stapedectomies using the Robinson vein graft technique that had been performed on six high-performance pilots diagnosed to be suffering from otosclerosis. All of them returned to full active duty following stapedectomy without any vestibular symptoms. Katzav et al concluded that it can be safe for fighter or test pilots to return to full flight status following stapedectomy. They also found that full flight status can be reinstated as soon as 3 months after stapedectomy without endangering flight safety.

House et al (2001) in their study sought to determine the prevalence of adverse auditory and/or vestibular sequelae in patients following stapedectomy. The authors mailed survey questionnaires to 2222 patients who had undergone stapedectomy at a single tertiary otologic referral center between 1987 and 1998. Of the initial 917 respondents, 208 (22.7%) had snorkeled, scuba-dived, or sky-dived following stapedectomy. One hundred forty of these patients responded to a second questionnaire detailing dive protocols, otologic symptoms, and their relationship to their diving activities. Of these 140 patients, 28 of them had scuba-dived or sky-dived. Four of the 22 scuba divers (18.1%) experienced otologic symptoms at the time of diving. These included otalgia on descent (3 of 22, 13.6%), tinnitus (1 of 22, 4.5%), and transient vertigo on initial submersion (1 of 22, 4.5%). One patient developed sudden sensorineural hearing loss and vertigo 3 months after scuba diving, which he related to noise exposure. This patient was subsequently found to have a perilymphatic fistula, which was repaired, and hearing was restored. Nine patients who sky-dived (22.2%) reported otologic symptoms during the dive. No significant diving-related long-term effects indicative of labyrinthine injury were seen in any of the 28 patients. The authors concluded that stapedectomy does not appear to increase the risk of inner ear barotrauma in scuba and skydivers. They reported that these activities may be pursued with relative safety following stapes surgery, provided adequate eustachian tube function has been established.

## STAPEDECTOMY FOLLOWING TYMPANOPLASTY

What is the incidence of otosclerosis in chronic otitis media? Is stapedectomy contraindicated in those patients suffering from chronic otitis media? Berenholz and colleagues (2001) reported an incidence of 0.3% (14 stapedectomies out of 4,678 over a 10-year period had had a tympanoplasty done prior to stapedectomy). In their series, all had a type 1 tympanoplasty. In other words, all the patients in this series had only a perforated tympanic membrane. An average period of 26 months elapsed between successful tympanoplasty and stapedectomy. No patients had simultaneous tympanoplasty and stapedectomy. Although all the perforations were fairly large, there was no correlation between the size of the perforation and postoperative results. Furthermore, there was no correlation between the number of months between the tympanoplasty and stapedectomy and poststapedectomy air-bone gap. In all of the patients, there was significant involvement of the stapes and footplate by tympanosclerosis.

The authors also noted a significant difference between the audiogram posttympanoplasty otosclerotic patient versus the pure otosclerotic patient. In those patients who have chronic otitis media and otosclerosis, the air-bone gap was larger. Berenholz et al concluded that the incidence of chronic otitis media in otosclerosis is rare. Patients with chronic otitis media and otosclerosis have a larger air-bone gap. Closure of the air-bone gap in these patients is significant but less than for those patients who have only otosclerosis without suffering from chronic otitis media. The results of stapedectomy are durable and reliable but not as good as for those patients who have suffered only from otosclerosis.

## CONTRAINDICATIONS

### Absolute Contraindication

All authors are in unanimous agreement that stapedectomy on the patient's only hearing ear is not recommended.

### Relative Contraindications

Contraindications to stapedectomy include the following:

1. Active middle ear or external ear infections. Once these conditions are treated and have resolved completely and satisfactorily, however, a stapedectomy can be performed after a suitable interval of time.

2. When the otosclerotic patient presents with symptoms of hydrops and has vertigo and tinnitus. These conditions should be completely controlled. Only when the patient is symptom free for a minimum period of 6 months can the patient be considered a suitable candidate for stapedectomy.

3. Stapedectomy is contraindicated in middle ear atelectasis, especially if the atelectasis is severe.

4. General medical diseases that cause the patient to be unfit to undergo surgery.

5. When the patient presents a positive Schwartze's sign, stapedectomy should not be done at that time. The patient should be given sodium fluoride and observed. Only when the Schwartze's sign has receded and the patient's disease has stabilized can the patient be considered fit to undergo surgery.

6. Surgery is contraindicated during pregnancy. Once pregnancy is over, a stapedectomy can be performed after a suitable interval of time.

7. Surgery is contraindicated in those whose professional activities put them at risk. Patients such as boxers, professional wrestlers, and those who indulge in severe physical strain should avoid having a stapedectomy done until they have given up such activities.

## PREOPERATIVE COUNSELING

All patients who are about to undergo a stapedectomy should be told about the pros and cons of stapedectomy. Patients should be told about the real risk of permanent sensorineural hearing loss, no matter how small the chance is of such an event occurring. They should be offered the opportunity of seeking alternative measures such as hearing aids and medical management of the problem.

Patients should be given detailed instructions that should be followed in the postoperative period. They should be advised against lifting heavy weights, to cough or sneeze without straining, and to avoid instrumenting the ear. Patients should be instructed to be alert and to report immediately any symptoms that might herald complications, such as vertigo, tinnitus, and hearing loss.

## PROCEDURE AND RECOMMENDATIONS

### Instruments and Equipment

The instruments used in stapedectomies are standard, with little variation (Fig. 10–1). Some surgeons, however, advocate using a speculum holder (Fig. 10–2). The advantage of the speculum holder is that this leaves the surgeon with both hands free to operate. On the other hand, some surgeons hold the speculum with the nondominant hand (i.e., in the case of right-handed surgeons, the speculum is held with the left hand), while the surgical maneuvers are performed with the dominant hand (Fig. 10–3).

A good operating microscope is an absolute necessity for the surgery (Fig. 10–4). The surgeon should start off at a low magnification and change to a higher magnification, especially when working on the footplate.

### Anesthesia

Most surgeons prefer local anesthesia, with the patient lightly sedated (Fig. 10–5). This gives the surgeon a chance to check if the patient's hearing improves immediately after the prosthesis has been inserted. The surgeon can check intraoperatively if the patient has any other symptoms, such as vertigo or tinnitus. In this way, the surgeon can be alerted immediately and take corrective action.

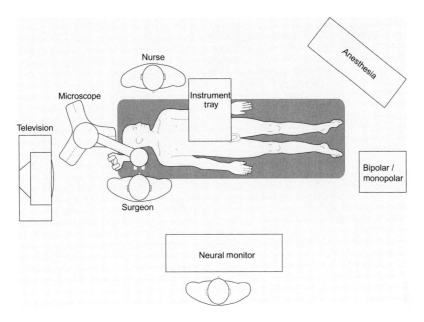

**Figure 10–1** Standard setup of an operating room for ear surgery.

General anesthesia avoids the situation of a struggling patient. The surgical steps can be gone through smoothly. The surgeon, however, is unable to check on the immediate impact of the surgery. The disadvantage of this situation is that if the prosthesis is too long and the patient experiences vertigo, then the surgeon may need to take the patient back into surgery to replace the prosthesis.

## Incision

Endaural incisions are useful if the canal is small or tortuous. They help widen the canal in such circumstances. Endomeatal incisions are good for large canals. They allow the surgeon to look comfortably into the middle ear while giving the surgeon a good exposure to the structures in the middle ear.

A local anesthetic (1 to 10,000 epinephrine solution in 2% xylocaine) is used to anesthetize the outer ear. The incision (Fig. 10–6) starts off at 6 o'clock, then curves back straight for about 1 cm away from the annulus. Another incision is made at 12 o'clock and should go straight back for about 1 cm. The two incisions should then join one another.

## Exposure of the Tympanic Cavity

The tympanomeatal flap is elevated, with care being taken not to tear the flap. The flap is elevated to the annulus from the 6 o'clock position to the 12 o'clock position (Fig. 10–7). Before elevating the annulus, meticulous hemostasis should be achieved. Should bleeding occur, it will obscure the surgeon's visibility of the crowded and delicate local anatomy. The annulus is then subluxated from its groove, and the middle ear cavity is entered (Fig. 10–8).

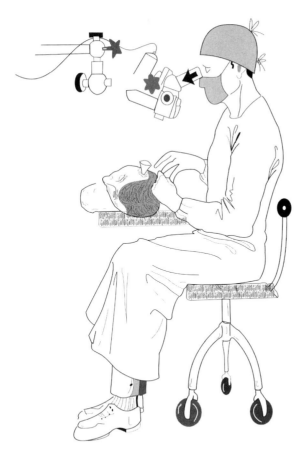

**Figure 10–2** Use of the speculum holder. (*From Schuknecht HF.* Stapedectomy. *Boston: Little, Brown; 1971. Used with permission.*)

The next steps are as follows:

1. The bony annulus is curetted away (Fig. 10–9). Curetting is complete (adequate) only when the entire stapedius tendon and the pyramidal eminence are seen. The long process of the incus should be seen in its entirety. Only then is curetting considered adequate. Some surgeons prefer to remove the bony annulus with a high-speed micromotor.

2. When removing the bony annulus, the chorda tympani will be encountered. The chorda tympani should be gently elevated from its entry into the middle ear all the way across the handle of the malleus. In this way, the chorda will not obstruct vision. Only if it is absolutely vital should the chorda be sacrificed. It is better to sacrifice the chorda than to stretch it. Most surgeons make efforts to preserve the chorda tympani.

3. The middle ear is entered and is now carefully inspected. All the ossicles are inspected for any possible abnormality. The oval window is also inspected to examine its appearance. Any other abnormalities,

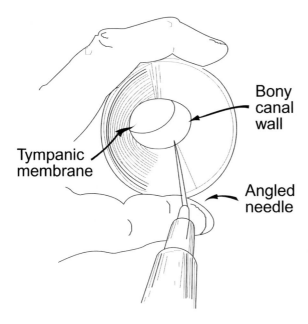

Bony
canal
wall

Tympanic
membrane

Angled
needle

**Figure 10–3** Using the dominant hand for surgery while the nondominant hand holds, steadies, and adjusts the speculum. (*From Schuknecht HF.* Stapedectomy. *Boston: Little, Brown; 1971. Used with permission.*)

such as an overhanging or dehiscent facial nerve and persistent stapedial artery, if present, are noted. The round window niche is also inspected.

4. The individual mobility of each ossicle is tested gently with a straight pick. First the malleus, then the incus, and finally the stapes are tested for mobility. It is important to rule out fixation of the malleus or fixation of the malleus and incus at this juncture. Once it is ascertained that only the stapes is fixed, a small control hole is created near the posterior crus.

5. The tendon of the stapes is divided (Fig. 10–10). This can be done with a scissors, sickle knife, or laser. The tendon should be divided near the pyramidal eminence. If the surgeon is reconstructing the stapedial muscle, it should be divided near its insertion into the stapes. As long a length of the muscle as possible should be preserved.

### Preserving the Stapedial Muscle

The Causse technique describes preserving the stapedial muscle. This is an attempt to replicate the physiological protective stabilizing effect of the stapes muscle on the prosthesis. Most conventional techniques do not reconstruct the stapedius muscle. Necrosis of the long process of the incus does not occur with reconstruction of the stapedius muscle. The Causse technique is known as stapedioplasty. The incidence of perilymph fistula is reported to be low with this technique. The disadvantage of this technique is that reclosure of the oval window is higher.

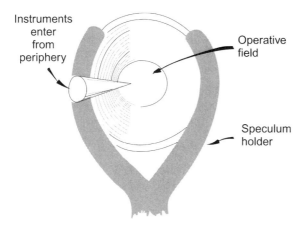

**Figure 10–4** Correct positioning of speculum holder and speculum. (*From Schuknecht HF.* Stapedectomy. *Boston: Little, Brown; 1971. Used with permission.*)

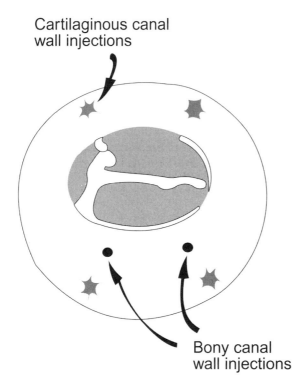

**Figure 10–5** Sites at which the local anesthetic should be injected. (*From Schuknecht HF.* Stapedectomy. *Boston: Little, Brown; 1971. Used with permission.*)

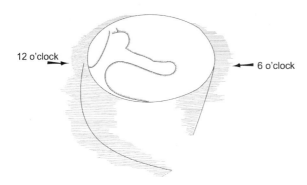

**Figure 10–6** The endomeatal incision. (*From Schuknecht HF.* Stapedectomy. *Boston: Little, Brown; 1971. Used with permission.*)

Colletti and Fiorino (1994) found that stapedectomy with reconstruction of the stapedius tendon has certain advantages and report superior results in an earlier article (Colletti et al 1988). The authors stated that stapedius muscle preservation (STP) has the lowest incidence of complications in their series (0.9%), compared with that of stapedius muscle section with small fenestra, where the complication rate was 4.5%, as well as with that of plain stapedectomy, where the complication rate was 10.1%. They claimed that STP maintained the blood supply to the lenticular process of the incus. It optimized the stabilization of the prosthesis, which in turn prevented migration of the prosthesis. Furthermore, STP maintained an adequate stiffness of the middle ear and conferred a "static" high pass filter to the reconstructed system. Colletti and Fiorino (1994) found that stapedotomy with preservation of the stapedius muscle is the method of choice. In their report on STP, Gierek and Bielecki (1999) found that there was no significant difference in those patients who had the stapedius muscle reconstructed versus those who had the stapedius sectioned.

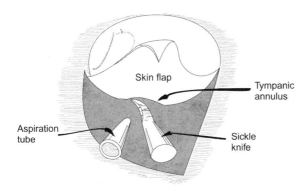

**Figure 10–7** Elevating the tympanomeatal flap. (*From Schuknecht HF.* Stapedectomy. *Boston: Little, Brown; 1971. Used with permission.*)

**99**

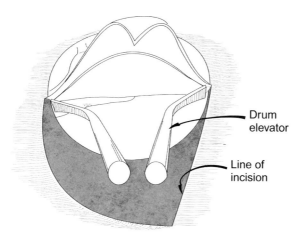

**Figure 10–8** Entering the middle ear. (*From Schuknecht HF.* Stapedectomy. *Boston: Little, Brown; 1971. Used with permission.*)

6. The incudostapedial joint is divided completely. This is done with a right-angled pick (Fig. 10–11).

7. The stapes is then fractured toward the promontory (Fig. 10–12). Great care should be taken at this stage because if the stapes is not fractured properly or if too much force is exerted, a floating footplate may result. Causse et al (1993) have described a special crura cutting scissors and lasers for this step of the surgery.

8. The mucosa over the footplate is excoriated (Fig. 10–13) along its entire length. This is an important step to prevent perilymph formation. Bleeding may occur at this time; this is controlled by Gelfoam application. This step requires patience. Should the surgeon be in a hurry to open

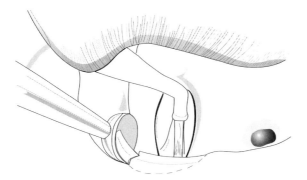

**Figure 10–9** Curetting the bony annulus to expose the stapes, the pyramidal eminence, and the stapedius tendon. (*From Friedman MD. Surgical management of otosclerosis: Primary stapedectomy surgery.* Operative Tech Otolaryngol Head Neck Surg. *1998;9(1):15. Used with permission.*)

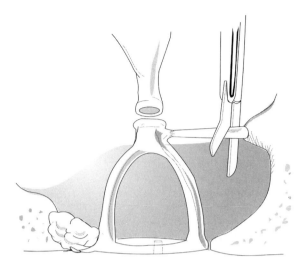

**Figure 10–10** Dividing the stapedius tendon. (*From Friedman MD. Surgical management of otosclerosis: Primary stapedectomy surgery. Operative Tech Otolaryngol Head Neck Surg. 1998;9(1):16. Used with permission.*)

the vestibule with bleeding still present, the blood will obscure his or her vision, and precise surgery will be impossible.

9. A measuring rule (Figs. 10–14, 10–15) is placed from the medial surface of the incus to the footplate, and the distance is measured. The average distance from the footplate to the undersurface of the incus is approximately 4.25 mm. Another 0.5 mm is added when selecting the

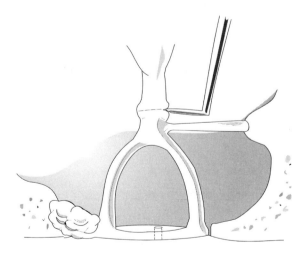

**Figure 10–11** Dividing the incudostapedial joint. (*From Friedman MD. Surgical management of otosclerosis: Primary stapedectomy surgery. Operative Tech Otolaryngol Head Neck Surg. 1998;9(1):15. Used with permission.*)

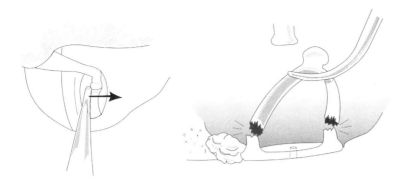

**Figure 10–12**   Fracturing the stapes superstructure. (*From Friedman MD. Surgical management of otosclerosis: Primary stapedectomy surgery.* Operative Tech Otolaryngol Head Neck Surg. *1998;9(1):16. Used with permission.*)

appropriate length of the prosthesis. The prosthesis should project 0.25 mm into the vestibule.

10. The control hole is widened (Fig. 10–16) to about 0.8 mm in a small fenestra stapedectomy. The fenestra should be placed in the posterior half of the footplate to avoid damage to the saccule and utricle. Sometimes a partial stapedectomy needs to be performed, and the posterior third of the footplate is removed (Figs. 10–17, 10–18). This should be done with a right-angled pick. The surgeon should not place the aspirator in the operating field once the vestibule has been opened. This is to avoid inadvertent aspiration of perilymph.

11. The oval window fenestra is covered with a connective tissue seal (Fig. 10–19). Both of this text's authors prefer to use perichondrium, which is

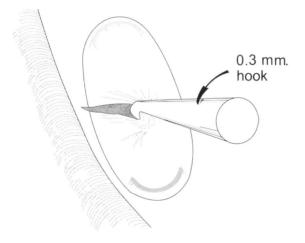

0.3 mm. hook

**Figure 10–13**   Removing the mucosa over the footplate. (*From Schuknecht HF.* Stapedectomy. *Boston: Little, Brown; 1971. Used with permission.*)

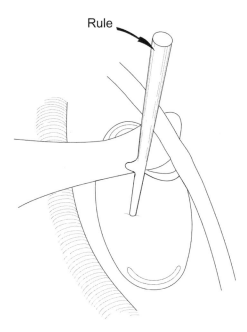

**Figure 10–14** Taking measurements from the long process of the incus to the footplate. (*From Schuknecht HF.* Stapedectomy. *Boston: Little, Brown; 1971. Used with permission.*)

easy to harvest, being near the operative site, and easy to handle. The disadvantage of using perichondrium rather than a vein graft seal is that vein grafts are much more elastic and springy, whereas perichondrium is stiffer.

**12.** The appropriate prosthesis is then placed.

## CHOOSING PROSTHESES

There are many prostheses available. The senior author has used the House wire prosthesis and the Robinson bucket handle prosthesis (Figs. 10–20, 10–21, 10–22). The junior author has used the Causse Teflon prosthesis (Fig. 10–23, 10–24, 10–25).

### Types of Prostheses Available

Various prostheses are available for stapedectomies (Fig. 10–26).

#### Robinson Prosthesis
The advantages of the Robinson prosthesis is that it does not require crimping and it is relatively easy to insert. The prosthesis is also self-centering. A narrow stem prosthesis is also available that can be used for posterior half footplate removal. This is a metal stem prosthesis designed to fit under the lenticular process of the incus.

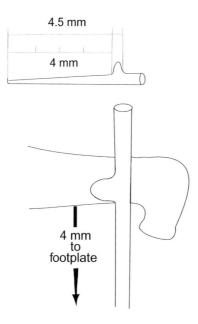

**Figure 10–15** Placing the rule on the undersurface of the incus. (*From Schuknecht HF.* Stapedectomy. *Boston: Little, Brown; 1971. Used with permission.*)

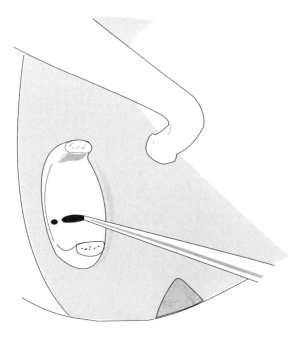

**Figure 10–16** Widening the control hole. (*From Friedman MD. Surgical management of otosclerosis: Primary stapedectomy surgery.* Operative Tech Otolaryngol Head Neck Surg. *1998;9():17. Used with permission.*)

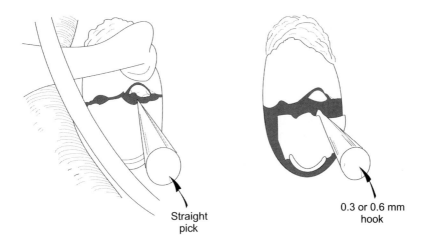

**Figure 10–17** Removing the posterior portion of the footplate for partial stapedectomy. (*From Schuknecht HF.* Stapedectomy. *Boston: Little, Brown; 1971. Used with permission.*)

### Causse Prosthesis

The Causse prosthesis is made of Teflon and is designed to attach to the long process of the incus. The Teflon ring is spread open, and the prosthesis is snapped onto the incus. Teflon has a long memory and does not require crimping. The prosthesis can be adjusted easily. This prosthesis can be used in small fenestra stapedectomy.

### Fisch/McGee Piston Prosthesis

The Fisch/McGee piston prosthesis consists of a malleable ribbon-like crook connected to a metal or Teflon stem. The crook is attached to the long process of the incus and must be crimped into position. One advantage of the prosthesis is that the distal end is scored; this makes it easy to check the

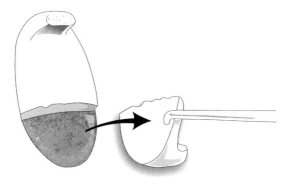

**Figure 10–18** Removal of the posterior portion of the footplate. (*From Friedman MD. Surgical management of otosclerosis: Primary stapedectomy surgery.* Operative Tech Otolaryngol Head Neck Surg. *1998;9(1):17. Used with permission.*)

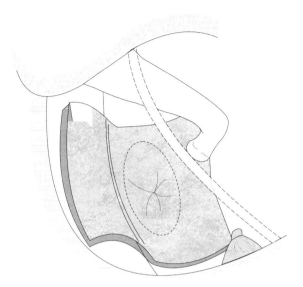

**Figure 10–19** Placement of a connective tissue seal over the fenestra. (*From Friedman MD. Surgical management of otosclerosis: Primary stapedectomy surgery.* Operative Tech Otolaryngol Head Neck Surg. *1998; 9(1):19. Used with permission.*)

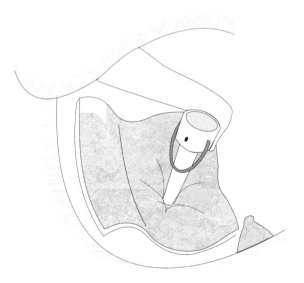

**Figure 10–20** Placing a Robinson bucket handle prosthesis. (*From Friedman MD. Surgical management of otosclerosis: Primary stapedectomy surgery.* Operative Tech Otolaryngol Head Neck Surg. *1998; 9(1):18. Used with permission.*)

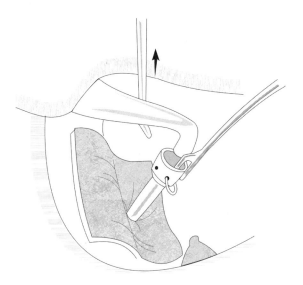

**Figure 10–21** Robinson prosthesis in the fenestra. (*From Friedman MD. Surgical management of otosclerosis: Primary stapedectomy surgery.* Operative Tech Otolaryngol Head Neck Surg. *1998;9(1):18. Used with permission.*)

exact length of the prosthesis that is required. The Fisch/McGee prosthesis can be used in small fenestra stapedectomy.

### House Wire Prosthesis

One end of the House wire prosthesis is shaped like a shepherd's crook (Fig. 10–27). At the other end is a loop. The crook is attached and crimped to the long process of the incus. The House prosthesis is technically more difficult to attach than other prostheses. It is used in total stapedectomy.

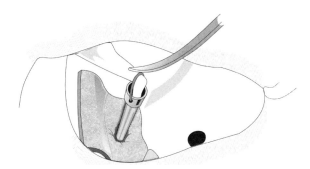

**Figure 10–22** Robinson prosthesis in place. (*From Friedman MD. Surgical management of otosclerosis: Primary stapedectomy surgery.* Operative Tech Otolaryngol Head Neck Surg. *1998;9(1):18. Used with permission.*)

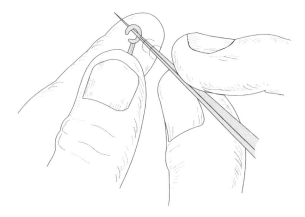

**Figure 10–23** Teflon prosthesis opened with a straight pick prior to placing it on the incus. (*From Friedman MD. Surgical management of otosclerosis: Primary stapedectomy surgery.* Operative Tech Otolaryngol Head Neck Surg. *1998;9(1):53. Used with permission.*)

## Failure Rates of Prostheses

Raske and colleagues (Raske et al 2001) reported on the long-term follow-up of patients who had undergone stapedectomy with the McGee stapes prosthesis. They reported on 170 stapedectomies (120 primary and 50 revision stapedectomies) from 1989 to 1999. The data (audiometric, clinical findings, and intraoperative findings) were analyzed and reported. Over a 10-year period, 11.2% of patients had failure of their initial air-bone gap closure with the McGee piston. Seventy-seven percent (10 out of 13 patients) of McGee pistons that failed were found to have the platinum ribbon displaced laterally from the incus and the piston pushed out of the fenestra.

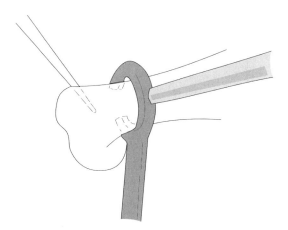

**Figure 10–24** Teflon piston placed on the incus. (*From Friedman MD. Surgical management of otosclerosis: Primary stapedectomy surgery.* Operative Tech Otolaryngol Head Neck Surg. *1998;9(1):54. Used with permission.*)

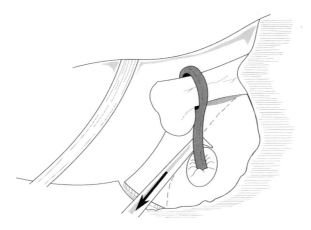

**Figure 10–25** Teflon piston in small fenestra. (*From Friedman MD. Surgical management of otosclerosis: Primary stapedectomy surgery.* Operative Tech Otolaryngol Head Neck Surg. *1998;9(1):54. Used with permission.*)

The failure rate was not significantly different ($p = .72$) from that in our patients who underwent placement of a Robinson cup prosthesis (9.5%), but the pattern of displacement was unique. Failures occurred earlier with the McGee piston (average time to failure 2.5 years) than with the Robinson cup (average time to failure 8.6 years). Raske et al concluded that the McGee piston was found to have a unique pattern of dislocation over time that is likely related to the malleable nature of the platinum ribbon and loosening of the crimped "shepherd's crook" over time.

Kos et al (2001) reported on their findings with Teflon wire prostheses. They analyzed the results of 604 primary stapedectomies performed between 1974 and 1997 using a 0.6 or 0.8 mm Schuknecht Teflon wire prosthesis.

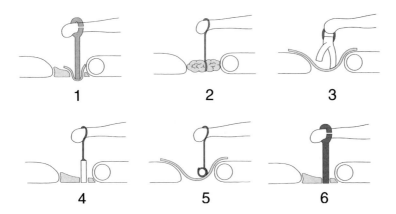

**Figure 10–26** Types of prostheses available. 1, teflon piston with vein graft used as a seal; 2, wire with fat; 3, posterior crus rotated (plainectomy); 4, teflon and wire; 5, wire with perichonchium seal interposed; 6, teflon piston placed through small finestra (stapedotomy) using blood as a seal. (*From Beales PH. Otosclerosis. Bristol: John Wright and Sons; 1981. Used with permission.*)

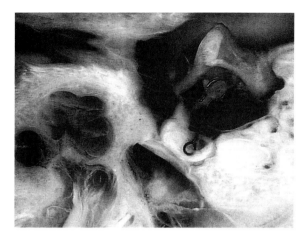

**Figure 10–27** Photomicrograph of a House wire stapedectomy prosthesis.

At follow-up (1 to 21 years; mean 7 years), the residual air-bone gap was 10 dB or less in 79% of the cases. Kos et al concluded that their results were comparable to those of other authors using various prostheses.

## Does the Weight of the Prosthesis Matter?

To answer this question, Bruijn et al (1999) compared the individual audiometric results obtained after using a gold or Teflon prosthesis. The gold prosthesis was the heavier of the two. In their retrospective study, Bruijn et al used a Teflon piston (Causse; Xomed Surgical Products, Jacksonville, FL) and a pure gold piston (K Piston; Heinz Kurz GmbH Medizintechnik, Düblingen, Germany). Retrospective analyses were carried out of the pre-surgery and postsurgery audiologic results obtained after primary stapedotomy by implantation of 62 Teflon pistons and 66 gold pistons. The results were compared according to mean values of several audiometric parameters. Additionally, individual audiograms were evaluated with the Amsterdam Hearing Evaluation Plots (AHEP). With this method, "unsuccessful" and "successful" inserted prosthesis could be recognized easily, and a more realistic comparison between prostheses was possible. Bruijn et al reported in their findings that, overall, the heavier gold prosthesis gave significantly larger gain in air conductive hearing at 2 kHz ($p < .05$) and in the speech frequency range of 0.5 to 2 kHz ($p < .05$). There were no significant intergroup differences in bone conduction and air-bone gap changes. An analysis of successfully implanted prostheses according to the AHEP criteria had consequences only in the improvement of air conduction thresholds. None of the intergroup differences were statistically significant. The authors concluded that the heavier gold piston gave more gain in the lower and mid-frequency range, and the lighter Teflon piston gave more gain in the high-frequency range, although none of the differences were significant.

Although changing the weight of the prosthesis in stapes surgery may have only a relatively small effect on the final hearing result, this effect may be significant if it contributes to approximately 5 dB more gain over other prostheses. It can be an influential factor in determining the type of prosthesis to be used in patients with mixed hearing losses because such a gain can be critical in changing the result from a nonserviceable hearing level to a serviceable one. In Bruijn et al's results, the mean hearing gain in the speech frequencies at 0.5 Hz, 1 kHz, and 2 kHz pure tone audiogram (PTA) differs 4.5 dB in favor of the gold piston and was statistically significant in the whole group of successfully and unsuccessfully implanted prostheses. After analyzing the results after exclusion of "unsuccessful" operations identified with the AHEP critieria, however, the intergroup difference was 3.1 dB and was not statistically significant.

Robinson (1974) performed a clinical comparative study between two prostheses with a difference in weight. He compared the results following stapedectomy. In his study, he used the Robinson stainless steel prosthesis (weight 12.5 mg) and the Robinson Teflon prosthesis (weight 3.3 mg). Better hearing results were obtained with the heavier stainless steel prosthesis in the low frequencies and in the higher frequency ranges. Furthermore, Robinson found that the rate of overclosures was much higher with the heavier stainless steel prosthesis.

## Does the Size of the Prosthesis Matter?

Fucci and colleagues (1998) examined 60 patients to determine if the diameter of the prosthesis contributed to hearing results. They used a 0.4 mm diameter Robinson prosthesis in one ear and a 0.6 mm Robinson prosthesis in the other ear of the same patient. The patients underwent bilateral stapedectomy. All patients had the same surgeon, the same length prosthesis (4 mm Robinson), the same oval window seal, and the same audiometric evaluation. A laser was not used for any patient. Audiologic assessment was carried out preoperatively, and at 1 month, 6 months, and 1 year postoperatively. This study was unique because the opposite ear of each patient was the basis for comparison, eliminating several patient variables. Fucci et al concluded that no differences were observed in the hearing results of 60 patients who had a 0.4 mm Robinson prosthesis in one ear and a 0.6 mm Robinson prosthesis in the other ear. All patients underwent a partial stapedectomy, a vein graft over the oval window, and a 4 mm long prosthesis. All patients had successful hearing results in both ears. The authors determined that a difference of 0.2 mm in prosthesis width had no significant effect on hearing results in a large fenestra stapedectomy. They now use a 0.4 mm prosthesis in all cases because a 0.6 mm prosthesis can occasionally be too wide for a narrow oval window niche.

This report is in contrast to a study by Sennaroglu et al (2001), who reported that the gain in air conduction levels was better with the use of 0.8 mm Teflon pistons than 0.6 mm Teflon pistons, particularly in the lower frequencies.

## What Is the Optimum Length of the Prosthesis That Should Be in the Fenestra?

The optimal length of the prosthesis in the fenestra should be approximately 0.1 to 0.2 mm below the fenestra (Lesinski 1998). Too long a prosthesis could result in vestibular symptoms and tinnitus, whereas too short a prosthesis could result in a conductive hearing loss. The prosthesis could migrate from the fenestra in the postoperative period.

## What Should an Ideal Prosthesis Be?

In their comparative electron microscopic study of the surface structure of gold, Teflon, and titanium stapes prostheses, Kwok et al (2001) concluded that the surface of the stapes prosthesis should show a certain roughness at the piston end to allow stable membrane attachment to the piston. The prosthesis should be roughened for better attachment or ossification in the loop area. It should have a band-shaped loop that is malleable enough to achieve a good attachment with the incus and should be stiff enough to prevent loosening of the band. Furthermore, the stiffness of the band should not cause an erosion of the long process of the incus. The transition zone from the piston to the loop area should be platform-shaped for better handling during surgery. The shaft should be long to prevent scar tissue from reaching the platform. The prosthesis should be of similar weight to the human stapes. The prosthesis diameter should be 0.4 mm. The material of the prosthesis should be biocompatible and corrosion resistant and should not cause allergic reactions.

13. Following placement of the prosthesis, the malleus is palpated, and the movement of the prosthesis is inspected. The tympanomeatal flap is repositioned.

14. The patient is gently aroused and asked if hearing has improved. The patient is also asked if vertigo or tinnitus is experienced. If the patient experiences sudden vertigo, this means that the prosthesis is too long, and the prosthesis may need to be replaced with one of an appropriate length. Some authors suggest checking the patient's hearing with a 512 Hz tuning fork.

15. The external auditory canal is packed with Gelfoam or with antibiotic ointment. A stitch is taken over the tragus from where the perichondrium has been harvested.

## POSTOPERATIVE CARE

Following surgery, the patient should be advised against violent movement in the first 24 hours. Slight dizziness may be experienced, but this usually subsides. Analgesics and antiemetics may be given. The patient is advised against straining. The following day, the patient is encouraged to be ambulatory.

## CAUSES OF FAILURE OF STAPEDECTOMY

Causes for reappearance of conductive hearing losses include migration of the prosthesis (Fig. 10–28). The prosthesis usually migrates to the edge of the fenestra until it loses contact, resulting in a conductive hearing loss. This is especially true if the prosthesis is loosely fitting around the incus.

Erosion or necrosis of the long process of the incus is another cause of reappearance of a conductive hearing loss (Fig. 10–28, 10–29). Lippy and Schuring (1974) recommend building up the long process of the incus with

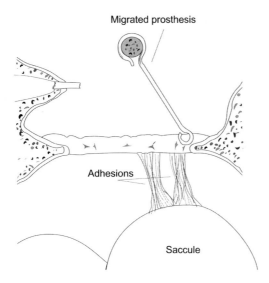

**Figure 10–28** A prosthesis that has migrated to the edge of the fenestra. (*From Friedman MD. Surgical management of otosclerosis: Revision stapedectomy surgery. Operative Tech Otolaryngol Head Neck Surg. 1998; 9(2):73. Used with permission.*)

ionomeric cement, whereas Sheehy (1982) recommends incus replacement prosthesis. Adhesions can cause restrictions of the movement of the incus and the prosthesis. At times the adhesions can cause the prosthesis to migrate to the edge of the fenestra.

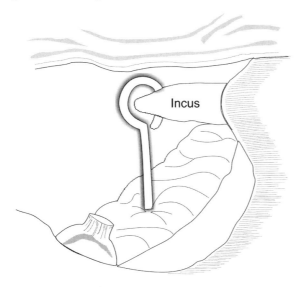

**Figure 10–29** Necrosis of the long process of the incus. (*From Friedman MD. Surgical management of otosclerosis: Revision stapedectomy surgery. Operative Tech Otolaryngol Head Neck Surg. 1998;9(2). Used with permission.*)

## WHO SHOULD PERFORM STAPEDECTOMIES?

If the answer were "Only experienced surgeons," then very few surgeons would perform stapedectomies. Many reports (Backhous et al 1993; Burns and Lambert 1996; Coker et al 1988; Handley and Hicks 1990; Levenson et al 1987; Shapir et al 1985) have acknowledged a learning curve in residency and among junior stapedectomy surgeons, as well as a diminishing pool of patients suffering from otosclerosis. A surgeon with a special interest and a fellowship in otology, no matter how junior, will obviously be at an advantage over the casual stapedectomy surgeon (Sargent 2002).

All those who undertake stapedectomy should be familiar with all the possible findings and nuances of stapedectomy surgery. Should they encounter difficulties, they should acknowledge their limitations and abandon surgery rather than proceed and cause a calamity. Only an experienced stapedectomy surgeon should do revision stapedectomies.

## PATIENT-PERCEIVED OUTCOMES FOLLOWING STAPEDECTOMY

Meyer and Megerian (2000) conducted a retrospective study of 29 patients who had undergone stapedectomy to evaluate how well their subjective perceptions of hearing improvement correlated with objective audiometric measurements. Patients expressed their assessment of hearing function by completing two versions of the Hearing Disability and Handicap Scale (HDHS). One version of the HDHS was based on patients' retrospective recollections of their hearing impairment prior to surgery, and the other reflected their assessment of their current function. Meyer and Megerian evaluated the HDHS data separately as well as in conjunction with pre- and postoperative audiometric findings. Following surgery, the group's mean pure tone average improved significantly from 58 to 27 dB; that is, the average patient had moderate to severe hearing loss preoperatively and only a mild hearing loss postoperatively. Significant improvement was also reflected in the difference between the mean pre- and postoperative HDHS scores, although some patients indicated that they experienced almost no improvement. Meyer and Megerian's overall findings indicated that there was a relationship between objective and subjective assessments of hearing improvements following surgery, but that it was weak. Although most patients perceived significant improvement, the degree of that perceived improvement cannot be predicted from pure tone audiogram. The authors concluded their study with the observation that a significant difference between audiometric findings and HDHS is useful in identifying patients who might benefit from additional counseling and/or aural rehabilitation.

## THE EFFECT OF STAPEDECTOMY ON HIGH FREQUENCIES AND SPEECH RECOGNITION

Meyer (1999) retrospectively analyzed 38 patients (40 ears) who had undergone stapedectomy. His results showed that preoperative and postoperative audiograms exhibited a down-sloping configuration toward the high frequencies. Stapedectomy resulted in a significant improvement ($p < .05$) from

500 to 4000 Hz in air conduction and 500 to 2000 Hz in bone conduction. Analysis of variance showed that age had no bearing on preoperative audiometric results ($p > .05$) for air conduction, bone conduction, and the air-bone gap. Postoperatively, results of younger patients (4 to 8 kHz air conduction, 4 kHz bone conduction) were better than those of older patients ($p < .05$), but the high-frequency range was still poorer than age-matched controls in the younger group. Meyer concluded that stapedectomy resulted in significant closure of the air-bone gap between 500 Hz and 4 kHz but failed to influence hearing above 4 kHz. Age appeared to be an important variable, with poorer results in the high-frequency range in older patients.

## CAN STAPEDOTOMY BE PERFORMED AS AN OUTPATIENT PROCEDURE?

Corvera and colleagues (1996) examined the issue of whether small fenestra stapedotomy could be performed in an outpatient setting. The traditional standard of care was for 1 or 2 days of hospitalization following stapedotomy. Outpatient stapedotomy can have benefits for both the patient and the institution (Dickins 1986; Dickins and Graham 1989). Corvera et al (1996) conducted this case-controlled study to see if physical activity would lead to displacement of the prosthesis or to perilymphatic fistula. They assumed that any complication occurring after the first 6 months could not be caused by the lack of postoperative rest. The authors examined, among other things, auditory gain and vertigo. They concluded that in their studied population of small fenestra stapedotomy, no increase in morbidity was noticed in patients who were part of the outpatient group as compared with the hospitalized group.

## REFERENCES

Albera R, Giordano L, Rosso P, Canale A. Surgery of otosclerosis in the elderly. *Aging Clin Exp Res (Milano)*. 2001;13(1)8–10.

Awengen DF. Change of bone conduction thresholds by total footplate stapedectomy in relation to age. *Am J Otolaryngol*. 1993;14:105–110.

Backhous DD, Coker NJ, Jenkins HA. Prospective study of resident performed stapedectomy. *Am J Otolaryngol*. 1993;14(5):451–454.

Berenholz LP, Lippy WH, Burkey JM, Schuring AG, Rizer FM. Stapedectomy following tympanoplasty. *J Laryngol Otolaryngol*. 2001;115(6):444–446.

Bruijn AJG, Tange RA, Dreschler WA. Comparison of stapes prostheses: A retrospective analysis of individual audiometric results obtained after stapedectomy by implantation of a gold and Teflon piston. *Am J Otolaryngol*. 1999;20:573–580.

Burns JA, Lambert PR. Stapedectomy in residency training. *Am J Otolaryngol*. 1996; 17(2):210–213.

Causse JB, Gherini S, Horn KL. Surgical treatment of stapes fixation by fiberoptic argon laser stapedectomy with reconstruction of the annular ligament. *Otol Clin N Am*. 1993;26:395–416.

Coker NJ, Duncan NO, Wright GL, Jenkins HA, Alford BR. Stapedectomy trends for the resident. *Ann Otol, Rhinol Laryngol*. 1988;97(2, pt 1):109–113.

Colletti V, Fiorino FG. Stapedotomy with stapedius tendon preservation: Technique and long term results. *Otolaryngol—Head Neck Surg*. 1994;111(3, pt 1):181–188.

Colletti V, Sittoni V, Fiorino FG. Stapedotomy with and without stapedius tendon preservation versus stapedectomy: Long term results. *Am J Otolaryngol.* 1988;9: 136–141.

Corvera G, Cespedes B, Ysunza A, Arrieta J. Ambulatory vs. in patient stapedectomy: a randomized twenty patient pilot study. *Otolaryngol—Head Neck Surg.* 1996;114(3)355–359.

De la Cruz A, Angeli S, Slattery WH. Stapedectomy in children. *Otolaryngol—Head Neck Surg.* 1999;120(4):487–492.

Dickins JR. Comparative study of otologic surgery in outpatient and hospital settings. *Laryngoscope.* 1986;96:774–785.

Dickins JR, Graham SS. Otologic surgery in the outpatient versus the hospital setting. *Am J Otolaryngol.* 1989;10:252–255.

Fucci MJ, Lippy WH, Schuring AG, Rizer FM. Prosthesis size in stapedectomy. *Otolaryngol—Head Neck Surg.* 1998;118(1):1–5.

Gierek T, Bielecki I. Hearing status after stapedectomy with preservation or cutting of stapedius tendon. *Otolaryngologia Polska.* 1999;53(2):179–181.

Handley GH, Hicks JN. Stapedectomy in residency: the UAB experience. *Am J Otolaryngol.* 1990;11(2):128–130.

House JW, Sheehy JL, Antunez JC. Stapedectomy in children. *Laryngoscope.* 1980; 90(11, pt 1):1804–1809.

House JW, Toh EH, Perez A. Diving after stapedectomy: Clinical experience and recommendations. *Otolaryngol—Head Neck Surg.* 2001;125(4)356–360.

Katzav J, Lippy WH, Shamiss A, Davidson BZ. Stapedectomy in combat pilots. *Am J Otolaryngol.* 1996;18(5):687–688.

Khalifa A, el Guindy A, Erfan F. Stapedectomy for far advanced otosclerosis. *J Laryngol Otol.* 1998;112(2):158–160.

Kos MI, Montandon PB, Guyot JP. Short and long term results of stapedotomy and stapedectomy with a Teflon wire prosthesis. *Ann Otol, Rhinol Laryngol.* 2001; 110(10):907–911.

Kwok P, Fisch U, Strutz J, Jacob P. Comparative electron microscopic study of the surface structure of gold, Teflon and titanium stapes prostheses. *Otol Neurotol.* 2001;22(5):608–613.

Lesinski GS. Revision surgery for otosclerosis: 1998 perspective. *Operative Tech Otolaryngol—Head Neck Surg.* 1998;9(2):72–81.

Levenson MJ, Belluci RJ, Grimes C, Ingerman M, Parisier SC. Otosclerosis surgery in a resident training program. *Arch Otolaryngol—Head Neck Surg.* 1987;113(1):29–31.

Lippy WH. Special problems of otosclerosis surgery. In: Brackmann DE, Shelton C, Arriaga MA, eds. *Otologic Surgery.* Philadelphia: WB Saunders; 1994:348–355.

Lippy WH, Burkey JM, Arkis PN. Word recognition score changes after stapedectomy for far advanced otosclerosis. *Am J Otolaryngol.* 1998;19(1):56–58.

Lippy WH, Burkey JM, Fucci MJ, Schuring AG, Rizer FM. Stapedectomy in the elderly. *Am J Otolaryngol.* 1996;17(6):831–834.

Lippy WH, Burkey JM, Schuring AG, Rizer FM. Short and long term results of stapedectomy in children. *Laryngoscope.* 1998;108(4, pt 1):569–572.

Lippy WH, Schuring AG. Prosthesis for the problem incus in stapedectomy. *Arch Otolaryngol.* 1974;100:237–239.

Lippy WH, Wingate J, Burkey JM, Rizer FM, Schuring AG. Stapedectomy revision in elderly patients. *Laryngoscope.* 2002;112(6):1100–1103.

Mann WJ, Amedee RG, Fuerst G, Tabb HG. Hearing loss a complication of stapes surgery. *Otolaryngol—Head Neck Surg.* 1996;115:324–328.

Meyer SE. The effect of stapes surgery on high frequency hearing in patients with otosclerosis. *Am J Otolaryngol.* 1999;20(1):36–40.

Meyer SE, Megerian CA. Patients perceived outcomes after stapedectomy for otosclerosis. *Ear, Nose Throat J.* 2000;79(11):846–848, 851–852.

Millman B, Giddings NA, Cole JM. Long term follow up of stapedectomy in children and adolescents. *Otolaryngol—Head Neck Surg.* 1996;115(1):78–81.

Murphy TP, Wallis DL. Stapedectomy in the pediatric patient. *Laryngoscope.* 1996;106(11):1415–1418.

Namyslowski G, Scierski W, Mrowka-Kata K, Bilinska-Pietraszek E. Stapedectomy in the treatment of otosclerosis in children. *Otolaryngologia Polska.* 2001;55(5): 521–525.

Raske M, Welling JD, Gillium T, Welling DB. Long term stapedectomy results with the McGee prosthesis. *Laryngoscope.* 2001;111(11, pt 1):2060–2063.

Robinson M. Stapes prosthesis: Stainless steel vs. Teflon. *Laryngoscope.* 1974;84: 1982–1995.

Ruckenstein MJ, Rafter KO, Montes M, Bigelow DC. Management of far advanced otosclerosis. *Otol Neurotol.* 2001;22(4):471–474.

Sargent EW. The learning curve revisited: Stapedotomy. *Otolaryngol—Head Neck Surg.* 2002;126(1):20–25.

Sennaroglu L, Unal OF, Sennaroglu G, Gursel B, Belgin E. Effect of Teflon piston diameter on hearing result after stapedotomy. *Otolaryngol—Head Neck Surg.* 2001; 124(3):279–281.

Shapir A, Ophir D, Marshak G. Success of stapedectomy performed by residents. *Am J Otolaryngol.* 1985;6(5):388–391.

Shea PF, Ge X, Shea JJ. Stapedectomy for far advanced otosclerosis. *Am J Otolaryngol.* 1999;20(4):425–429.

Sheehy JL. Stapedectomy: incus bypass procedures. A report of 203 operations. *Laryngoscope.* 1982;92:258–262.

Szymanski M, Siwiec H, Golabek W, Morshed K. Short and long term results of stapedectomy in children. *Ann Universitatatis Mariae Curie Sklodowska—Sectio'd medicina (Poland).* 2001;56:412–416.

Vartiainen E. Surgery in the elderly patient with otosclerosis. *Am J Otolaryngol.* 1995; 16:536–538.

# Chapter *11*

# Obliterative Otosclerosis

Obliterative otosclerosis involves total obscuration of the oval window and its margins (Fig. 11–1). It is thought to be evidence of very advanced otosclerosis. Young patients are especially at risk, particularly when active, aggressive otosclerosis develops around puberty. Obliteration of the round window is less common, and total obliteration is rare. When the round window is obliterated, however, the patient usually has an accompanying sensorineural hearing loss.

Obliterative otosclerosis can occur within the vestibule as well. Involvement of the labyrinthine vestibule and cochlea aqueduct causes the cochlea to degenerate, with accompanying profound sensorineural hearing loss. Obliterative otosclerosis is very uncommon in unilateral otosclerosis.

## PATHOLOGY

Causse et al (1991) reported that obliterative otosclerosis is caused by the same immunoenzymatic process at work in cochlear otosclerosis. In the early stages of obliterative otosclerosis, thin osteoid lamellae are found in the deep part of the highly vascularized mucoperiosteum of the fissula ante fenestram. Once the disease advances, however, the stapes superstructure and its crura are eventually buried in the extension of otosclerotic bone that fills the oval window niche. Bone thickness in the obliterated oval window niche varies from 0.5 mm to more than 2.0 mm (Gristwood 1966).

Early attempts to drill out the obliterated footplate were accompanied by severe sensorineural hearing loss (Guilford 1963). Reclosure of the drilled-away footplate was reported in 50% of cases by House (1962). Some authors (e.g., Cody et al 1967) even considered the obliterated footplate as a reason to abandon stapedectomy.

## INCIDENCE

Gristwood (1966) reported a 12.5% incidence of obliterated footplates in his series, noting that cases of obliterative otosclerosis were almost invariably diagnosed during adolescence and were associated with the presence of aggressive disease. He found it impossible to predict before surgery on the basis of audiometry and clinical findings that an obliterated footplate awaited

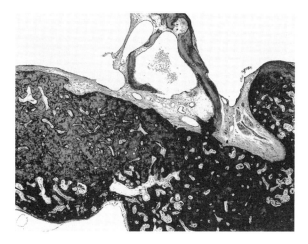

**Figure 11–1**  Photomicrograph of an obliterated footplate.

the surgeon. Gristwood attributed the high incidence of obliterated footplates in his series to the low levels of sodium fluoride in drinking water. It is interesting to note that all authors agree that obliterated footplates are found in adolescents and young adults usually at puberty, between the ages of 12 and 15 years. Gristwood and Venables (1983) reported that they found no strong evidence that pregnancy increases the progression of obliterative otosclerosis.

Other authors (Farrior 1981; Gristwood and Venables 1975; Shambaugh 1963) have quoted an incidence of obliterative otosclerosis ranging from 7 to 11% in their series. Amedee and Lewis (1987), however, quoted a figure of 20% in their series. Hurtado Garcia and colleagues (1995) reported a figure of 6.2% in their series. Ayache et al (1999) reported an incidence of 4.7% in their series and noted that there was a 50% chance that obliterative otosclerosis would be a bilateral finding.

Raman et al (1991) reported the following in their analysis of 420 consecutive cases of obliterative otosclerosis. The proportion of truly obliterated cases was 33.09%. The male to female ratio was 1.48 males per 1.0 female. In the nonobliterated cases, the ratio of male to female was 1.34:1.00. The mean age at onset was 19.14 years; in the nonobliterated cases, it was 25.60. This was found to be statistically significant ($p > .001$). In the nonobliterated cases, the age at onset was 30.86 and was not found to be as statistically significant.

## TYPES OF OBLITERATED FOOTPLATES

### Truly Obliterated Footplate

In the case of a truly obliterated footplate, the footplate is thickened and is later replaced by a massive otosclerotic focus (Fig. 11–2A). The boundaries of the footplate cannot be identified, and there is no delineation present to indicate the margins of the footplate. The crura of the footplate are covered

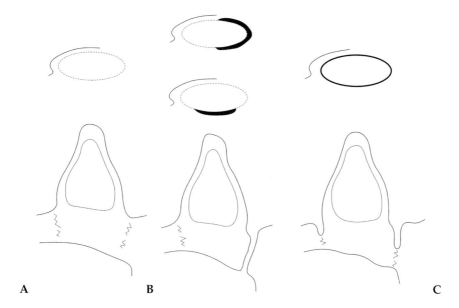

**Figure 11–2** Schematic representation of an obliterated footplate. **(A)** The footplate (dotted lines) is truly obliterated and cannot be distinguished from the surrounding bone. **(B)** The footplate is partly obliterated with a line of delineation (dark lines). **(C)** Spuriously obliterated footplate. The dark lines indicate apparent delineation of the footplate. *(From Beales PH. Otosclerosis. Bristol: John Wright and Sons; 1981. Used with permission.)*

and sometimes buried by the massive otosclerotic focus. The otosclerotic bone may be up to 2.5 mm thick.

## Partly Obliterated Footplate

A partly obliterated footplate occurs in approximately 4.6% of cases. The footplate is diffusely thickened; however, a rim of delineation can be identified (the rim may not be completely identifiable in the entire dimension of the footplate) (Fig. 11–2B).

## Spuriously Obliterated Footplate

The incidence of a spuriously obliterated footplate (Fig. 11–2C) is approximately 0.5%. In this situation, a surrounding rim is seen in the presence of a solid, thick footplate. It only becomes clear that the delineation is false when the surgeon tries to remove the footplate and fails because the footplate is thicker than anticipated.

## Biscuit Footplate

The biscuit, or "rice grain," footplate is diffusely thickened, while retaining a clear, well-delineated rim and an intact annular ligament. The surgeon should operate with caution in these situations, for it is easy for this kind of footplate to become dislodged.

## Crowded Oval Window Niche

In a crowded oval window niche, the oval window is crowded by the otosclerotic focus. A slitlike opening is all that is seen. The footplate, however, may be relatively thinner than a truly obliterated footplate. The overhanging bone should be removed with care before addressing the footplate.

## ROUND WINDOW OBLITERATION

As stated earlier, it is rare for the round window to be obliterated completely. It is not uncommon, however, to find the round window narrowed. Following the oval window, the round window is the second most common site at which otosclerosis occurs. The incidence of round window obliteration ranges from about 0.5 to 1.0%, as reported in the literature (Ginsberg et al 1978; Shea and Farrior 1987), although Causse et al (1991) reported that round window obliteration occurs only in approximately 1 in 250 cases. Preoperatively early onset of hearing loss, either in childhood or in adolescence, and a strong family history of otosclerosis are usually associated with obliteration of the round window.

Obliteration of the round window has a sensorineural component as opposed to a conductive element, as seen with obliteration of the oval window (Wiet et al 1993). Round window closure is thought not to contribute to hearing loss until the niche is completely obliterated. Even if there remains a small opening, it is thought to be adequate for vibratory motion of the cochlear fluids between the round and oval windows. Obliterated round windows should not be drilled out, as this leads to profound sensorineural hearing losses (Causse et al 1983). Delayed round window closure can occur following stapedectomy for far advanced otosclerosis (Mawson 1975). Should round window obliteration occur, some surgeons consider this to be an indication for sodium fluoride therapy (Shea and Farrior 1987).

## CAN AN OBLITERATED FOOTPLATE BE DIAGNOSED PRIOR TO SURGERY?

Obliterative otosclerosis cannot be diagnosed on the basis of clinical and audiometric evaluation. In the past, it was diagnosed only as a finding during surgery. Recent advances in CT scanning, however, can help diagnose an obliterated footplate.

The parameters on which a diagnosis of obliterated footplate can be made are as follows:

1. Early hearing impairment in teenagers and young adults

2. A positive Schwartze's sign

3. Bilateral rapid progression of hearing impairment (especially in the air-bone gap in young patients)

4. Low compliance in tympanometry

5. CT scan findings

When all these factors exist in the patient in whom otosclerosis is thought to be present, the surgeon should presume that an obliterated footplate is present.

## MANAGEMENT OF THE OBLITERATED FOOTPLATE

### Medical Treatment

Sodium fluoride therapy can slow or arrest the progression of an ongoing obliterated footplate. This is essential, especially when Schwartze's sign is positive. However, the treatment of an obliterated footplate is surgery (stapedectomy). A dosage of 25 to 50 mg is advised for 6 months prior to surgery. Fluoride treatment reduces the difficulty of surgery to a certain extent. If an obliterated footplate is discovered during surgery, however, sodium fluoride can still be given in the postoperative period. Postoperatively, the dosage given is usually 25 mg and can be tapered off to 5 mg.

### Surgery

The safest surgery for an obliterated footplate is often considered the small fenestra surgery. Nadol (2001), however, recommended a large fenestra so that this will accommodate the possibility of new bone formation and thus prevent failure of the primary stapedectomy. If the footplate is soft and friable, it is possible to make an opening of at least 1 mm in diameter. If the bone is hard, it may be necessary to use a micromotor and drill out the bone (Fig. 11–3). Lasers have added a new dimension of safety and convenience to surgery on an obliterated footplate.

If the footplate is to be drilled out, the drill bit should be turned slowly so as not to generate heat or prematurely enter the vestibule. The vestibule should be blue lined where a thin shelf of bone covers the vestibule. When the vestibule is blue lined, the fenestra can be created in the usual way.

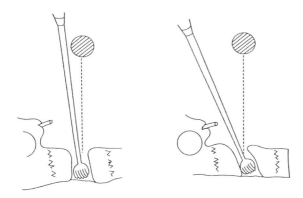

**Figure 11–3** Drill-out of the obliterated footplate. *(From Beales PH.* Otosclerosis. *Bristol: John Wright and Sons; 1981. Used with permission.)*

The piston selected must be long enough to extend beyond the otosclerotic focus. Gristwood (1966) noted that the thickness of the obliterated footplate varied from 0.5 to over 2.0 mm, so a longer piston was needed. He used a slim piston and sealed the fenestra with a connective tissue seal. No perilymphatic fistulae were seen in his series.

Causse et al (1991) recommended that late surgery in obliterative cases is safer than surgery performed before complete fixation of the footplate has taken place because this avoids excessive mobilization of labyrinthine fluids. They also found that the use of the long piston without the use of a vein graft seal was risky, having as its attendant risk a perilymphatic fistula. Causse et al reported that a longer piston may actually reach the saccule and traumatize it. There is also increased risk of reclosure if only a small channel is created in the foci on a large piece of bone. Furthermore, there is a great risk of bleeding into the vestibule if there is no seal interposed between the contents of the vestibule and the prosthesis.

Nadol (2001) noted that obliteration of the round window is the cause of failure of primary stapedectomy. Han et al (1997) noted similar findings in their series. Nadol wrote that in none of the cases of his series was there mention of the status of the round window at the time of surgery; the surgeon had overlooked this possibility. Therefore, Nadol recommended that at the time of surgery, whether it be primary or revision stapedectomy, the patency of the round window should be noted and documented. If noted, it should be drilled out carefully.

## RESULTS

Causse et al (1991) reported similar results in obliterated and nonobliterated cases. They found no incidence of sensorineural hearing loss following surgery on an obliterated footplate. No other problems such as dizziness, tinnitus, or facial palsy were found in their series.

## RECLOSURE (REOBLITERATION OF THE FOOTPLATE AND OTHER ASSOCIATED COMPLICATIONS)

Sensorineural hearing loss is significantly higher in obliterated footplates, especially when a drill-out procedure is required (House 1963). Regrowth or reclosure of the footplate occurs because of new bone growth. This new bone is different from otosclerotic bone and is not an otosclerotic focus (Linthicum 1980; Nadol 2001). Nadol (2001) considers it to be reparative bone.

Sheehy et al (1981) reported an incidence of 9% of reclosure by this reparative bone that returns to obliterate the footplate once again, thus resulting in failure of stapedectomy. Derlacki (1985) reported an incidence of zero reclosure, while Glasscock et al (1987) reported an incidence of 8%. In a series by Derlacki (1985), 50% of cases had partial reclosure, and the other half had total reclosure. Glasscock et al (1987) noted in their series that there was partial reclosure. Reclosure commonly occurs within 1 year of the primary stapedectomy. Wiet et al (1993) and Crabtree et al (1980) reported that sodium fluoride given at the time of primary stapes surgery when the obliterated footplate is first discovered serves to prevent regrowth.

## WHAT SHOULD THE SURGEON DO WHEN A RECLOSURE OCCURS AFTER PRIMARY STAPES SURGERY WHEN AN OBLITERATED FOOTPLATE HAS BEEN ENCOUNTERED?

Sheehy et al (1981) reported that when they attempted to drill out the reclosure, 8 of 17 patients (47%) developed a sensorineural hearing loss, of which 3 developed a profound sensorineural hearing loss. Derlacki (1985) and Shea (1963) advised against drilling out the reclosed footplate for this results in sensorineural hearing loss. Wiet et al (1993) recommended a high-resolution CT scan when a reclosure of an obliterated footplate is suspected following primary stapes surgery.

Gherini et al (1990) reported excellent results with the use of a fiberoptic, handheld argon laser when dealing with an obliterated footplate. They reported 10 cases where the fiberoptic argon laser was used and small fenestra stapedectomy was performed. Closure of the air-bone gap was seen in all patients. Postoperatively, there was no sensorineural hearing loss, vertigo, or facial weakness.

Cases of reclosure by new bone should be treated with caution. Hearing aids as a viable alternative should be given serious consideration.

## COMMENTS

Total footplate removal causes the otosclerotic focus to regrow, resulting in reobliteration. In obliterated footplates, the new bone that grows once again to obliterate the footplate is not otosclerotic bone but new bone that regrows probably in reparation to surgical trauma. Hence Nadol (2001) recommended a large fenestra stapedectomy when faced with an obliterated footplate. Reclosure of the footplate can occur even if a small fenestra stapedectomy is performed.

Obliterated footplates are usually found in young adults and teenagers. Rapid and early onset hearing loss in this age group usually indicates the possibility of an obliterated footplate. Obliteration is usually associated with bilateral otosclerosis, not unilateral otosclerosis. Obliterated footplates are usually discovered during surgery. In the active aggressive phase, sodium fluoride can be prescribed. Obliterated footplates are associated with a high incidence of failure due to reclosure of the fenestra by new bone. This bone is different from otosclerotic bone.

Large fenestra stapedectomy is one method of dealing with this problem. The introduction of lasers has served to provide a relatively atraumatic tool (as compared to a microdrill) when dealing with this problem. Redrilling of the footplate that has undergone reclosure following primary stapedectomy is associated with a high incidence of sensorineural hearing loss. Sodium fluoride therapy is indicated for these patients. The treatment of choice is still surgery.

## Congenital Footplate Fixation

Congenital footplate fixation is usually unilateral and is diagnosed in late childhood or adolescence. Unlike adolescent otosclerosis, the hearing loss is nonprogressive and has been present since birth. If the condition is bilateral, speech acquisition will be affected and the cause detected early. If it is unilateral, however, the conductive deafness will most likely be detected in late childhood or adolescence. The audiometric configuration can be identical to that of otosclerosis, including the presence of Carhart's notch. A perilymphatic fistula may be anticipated in patients with congenital footplate fixation (Glasscock 1973).

Dornhoffer et al (1995) and Hohmann and Dornhoffer (1995) reported on their experience in dealing with congenitally fixed footplates. They acknowledged at the outset that cerebrospinal fluid (CSF) and perilymph gushers are associated with this condition. The authors performed stapedectomy on 10 ears for congenitally fixed footplates. They did not encounter perilymph gushers, and none of the patients experienced a profound sensorineural hearing loss. All but one of the cases resulted in closure of the air-bone gap at the speech frequencies to within 20 dB, with the average air-bone gap being 11.2 dB. Minor congenital abnormalities of the stapes superstructure were seen in three of the cases. The authors reported that perilymph gushers in congenitally fixed footplates occurred almost exclusively in males.

Most otologists recommend leaving a congenital fixed footplate alone because of the high association of CSF/perilymph gushers and the accompanying profound sensorineural hearing loss that results. Beales (1981) reported success in mobilization of the footplate. There is no mention if the footplate refixed postoperatively, however.

## References

Amedee RG, Lewis ML. Obliterative otosclerosis. *Laryngoscope.* 1987;97(8 pt 1): 922–924.

Ayache D, Sleiman J, Plouin-Gaudon I, Klap P, Elbaz P. Obliterative otosclerosis. *J Laryngol Otol.* 1999;113(6):512–514.

Beales PH. Clinical features and diagnosis. In: *Otosclerosis.* Bristol: John Wright and Sons; 1981:25.

Causse JB, Causse JR, Wiet RJ. Special conditions in otosclerosis surgery. In: Wiet JR, Causse JB, Shambaugh GE, Causse JR, eds. *Otosclerosis (Otospongiosis).* American Academy of Otolaryngology—Head and Neck Surgery Foundation; Alexandria, Va; 1991:134–139.

Causse JB, Causse JR, Wiet RJ, Yoo TJ. Complications of stapedectomies. *Am J Otolaryngol.* 1983;4:275–280.

Cody DTR, Hallberg OE, Simonton KN. Stapedectomy for otosclerosis: Some causes of failure. *Arch Otolaryngol.* 1967;85:184–189.

Crabtree JA, Britton BH, Powers WH. An elevation of revision stapes surgery. *Laryngoscope.* 1980;90:224–227.

Derlacki EL. Revision stapes surgery: Problems with some solutions. *Laryngoscope.* 1985;95:1047–1053.

Dornhoffer JL, Helms J, Hoehmann DH. Stapedectomy for congenital fixation of the stapes. *Am J Otolaryngol.* 1995;16(3):382–386.

Farrior B. Contraindications to small hole stapedectomy. *Ann Otol, Rhinol Laryngol.* 1981;90:636–639.

Gherini SG, Horn KL, Bowman CA, Griffin G. Small fenestra stapedectomy using a fiberoptic handheld argon laser in obliterative otosclerosis. *Laryngoscope*. 1990; 11(2):1276–1282.

Ginsberg I, Hoffman SR, Stinziano GD, et al. Stapedectomy: In depth analysis of 2405 cases. *Laryngoscope*. 1978;88:1999–2016.

Glasscock ME. Stapes gusher. *Arch Otolaryngol*. 1973;98:81–82.

Glasscock ME, McKennan KX, Levine SC. Revision stapedectomy surgery. *Otolaryngol Head Neck Surg*. 1987;96:141–148.

Gristwood RE. Obliterative otosclerosis. *J Otolaryngol Soc Aust*. 1966;2:40–48.

Gristwood RE. Obliterative otosclerosis: An analysis of the clinical and audiometric findings. *J Laryngol*. 1996;80:115–120.

Gristwood RE, Venables WN. Otosclerosis of the oval window niche. *J Laryngol Otol*. 1975;89:1185–1217.

Gristwood RE, Venables WN. Pregnancy and otosclerosis. *Clin Otolaryngol*. 1983;8: 205–210.

Guilford F. Panel on footplate pathology, techniques and prognosis. *Arch Otolaryngol*. 1963;78:520–526.

Han WW, Incesulu A, McKenna MJ, et al. Revision stapedectomy: Intraoperative findings, results and review of literature. *Laryngoscope*. 1997;107:1185–1192.

Hohmann D, Dornhoffer J. Stapedectomy in congenital stapes fixation. *HNO*. 1995;43(2):65–69.

House HP. Footplate surgery in otosclerosis. *J Laryngol*. 1962;76:73.

House HP. Early and late complications of stapes surgery. *Arch Otolaryngol*. 1963; 78:606–613.

Hurtado Garcia JF, Lopez-Rico JJ, Talavera Sanchez J, Aracil Montesinos A. Obliterative otosclerosis. *Acta Otorhinolaryngologica Espanola*. 1995;46(3):171–174.

Linthicum FH. Histologic evidence of the causes of failure in stapes surgery. *Ann Otol, Rhinol Laryngol*. 1980;2:67–77.

Mawson SR. Management of complications of stapedectomy. *J Laryngol Otol*. 1975; 89:1445–1449.

Nadol JB. Histopathology of residual and recurrent conductive hearing loss after stapedectomy. *Otol Neurotol*. 2001;22(2):162–169.

Raman R, Masthew J, Idikula J. Obliterative otosclerosis. *J Laryngol Otol*. 1991; 105(11):899–900.

Shambaugh GE. Cochlear pathology after stapes surgery. *Arch Otolaryngol*. 1963;78: 214–219.

Shea JJ. Complications of the stapedectomy operation. *Ann Otol, Rhinol Laryngol*. 1963;72:1109–1123.

Shea JJ. How I do primary and revision stapedectomy. *Am J Otolaryngol*. 1994; 15(1)71–73.

Shea JJ, Farrior JB. Stapedectomy and round window closure. *Laryngoscope*. 1987; 97:10–12.

Sheehy JL, Nelson RA, House HP. Revision stapedectomy: A review of 258 cases. *Laryngoscope*. 1981;91:43–51.

Wiet RJ, Harvey SA, Bauer GP. Complications in stapes surgery. *Otolaryngol Clin N Am*. 1993;26(3):471–490.

# Chapter *12*

# Poststapedectomy Perilymph Fistulae

A perilymph fistula is one of the most common causes of sensorineural hearing loss following stapedectomy. It is thought that perilymph fistulae occur because of inadequate closure of the fenestra in the footplate by the seal, too long a prosthesis, or possibly increased perilymph pressure. The diagnosis and treatment of this condition are vital, because it has the potential to cause irreversible profound sensorineural hearing loss and puts the patient at risk of developing meningitis. Newlands (1976) reported on a patient who developed acute otitis media, labyrinthitis, and meningitis 16 months following stapedectomy. Poststapedectomy carries an increased risk of labyrinthitis and meningitis. Should labyrinthitis occur with or without meningitis, fistula repair must be taken as soon as the infection has been eliminated (Matz et al 1968).

Lewis (1961) described perilymph fistula, observing that the polyethylene strut caused perilymph to leak into the middle ear. Perilymph fistulae have been observed with all types of stapes surgeries and with all techniques.

## SIGNS AND SYMPTOMS OF PERILYMPH FISTULA

The most common symptoms are fluctuating sensorineural hearing loss, roaring tinnitus, and vertigo accompanied by fullness in the ear. These symptoms are also associated with endolymphatic hydrops. The key to making a diagnosis of perilymph fistula, however, is that it occurs following stapedectomy. If it occurs immediately following surgery, the diagnosis of perilymph fistula is obvious. This is termed *primary* or *early perilymph fistula*. If instead symptoms occur long after stapedectomy, then establishing a diagnosis of perilymph fistula may not be that easy. This is termed *delayed* or *secondary perilymph fistula*.

## INCIDENCE

Perilymph fistulae account for 9 to 10% of failures of stapedectomies (Crabtree et al 1980; Derlacki 1985; Glasscock et al 1987). On the other hand, Feldman and Schuknecht (1970) analyzed 154 revision stapedectomies and reported that perilymph fistulae were found in just 5 cases. The incidence of perilymph fistulae as a cause of failure in stapedectomy is approximately the same for both short- and long-term follow-up (Glasscock et al 1987).

## EARLY (PRIMARY) PERILYMPH FISTULA

Stapedectomy by necessity involves the creation of a fistula for the insertion of the prosthesis. The primary perilymph fistula occurs when the fistula created at the time of surgery persists and fails to seal off the vestibule from the middle ear. This can occur immediately after surgery, and symptoms can persist for days or weeks.

### Signs and Symptoms

The typical symptoms consist of hearing loss, tinnitus, and vertigo. Because these symptoms are also typical of endolymphatic hydrops, an early perilymph fistula can be confused with endolymphatic hydrops.

The most common symptom in some series is vertigo, whereas in others the most common symptom is a drop or a fluctuation in hearing (Wiet et al 1993). Harrison and colleagues (1967) reviewed 46 cases of poststapedectomy perilymph fistulae and found hearing loss or fluctuating hearing loss to be the most common symptom in 87% of cases. Moon (1970) examined 49 cases of poststapedectomy perilymph fistulae and found that 71% of cases with primary fistulae, and 78% of cases with secondary perilymph fistulae, presented with hearing loss as their chief complaint. Moon also reported that a pure sensorineural hearing loss is the most common type of loss in both primary and secondary fistulae. On occasion, however, mixed hearing losses and pure conductive hearing losses can occur as a symptom of perilymph fistula. Goodhill (1967) emphasized that a perilymph fistula may present only as a fluctuating or persistent conductive hearing loss. He postulated that the ratio of the transducer effect of the prosthesis to the perilymph spillage effect is less than ideal in such patients, thus accounting for their symptoms.

Vertigo may result from semicircular canal disturbances that then result in rotatory vertigo, or it may have a utricular origin, which results in a sense of falling down. Harrison et al (1967) found that 35% of their patients complained of vertigo, and 39% had a sensation of imbalance. Moon (1970) found that 77% of primary fistulae and 61% of secondary fistulae caused disequilibrium.

Tinnitus was found in 28% of patients, as reported by Harrison et al (1967). Moon (1970) found tinnitus to be present in 45% of patients who had a perilymph fistula.

The signs and symptoms vary with the size of the leak. Large fistulae result in rapid hearing loss, tinnitus, and vertigo. Morrison (1984) noted that such large fistulae accompanied technical difficulties by the operating surgeon at the time of stapedectomy. Fluctuation in hearing loss is unlikely to be a feature in such a situation. In early perilymph fistulae, when the leak is small, the hearing loss may initially appear as a conductive hearing loss; then has a sensorineural component; then progresses to a total sensorineural hearing loss. When such a fistula is repaired late, the hearing does not

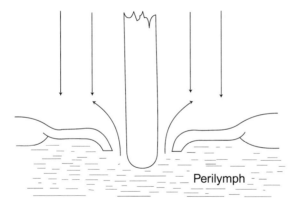

Perilymph

**Figure 12–1** A prosthesis without an adequate oval window seal creates a perilymph fistula. *(Adapted from Beales PH. Otosclerosis. Bristol: John Wright and Sons; 1981. Used with permission.)*

improve, although vertigo may resolve. When a minute fistula is present, the only evidence of the fistula is failure of a good closure of an air-bone gap, mild fluctuation in hearing, and a small decrease in speech discrimination scores.

## Cause of Primary Perilymph Fistula

Improperly sealed oval window fenestrae are the most likely cause of such fistulae (Fig. 12–1). Goodhill (1967) stated that if a mucosal seal does not hermetically seal off the vestibule from the middle ear at the time of surgery, then the chances of such a fistula forming are high. Failure to reflect the mucoperiosteal flaps may allow the lacerated edges of tissue to extend down into the vestibule and prevent formation of a new endosteal membrane at the level of the oval window. A prosthesis that is too long will also prevent the fistula from sealing off.

Numerous studies (Sheehy et al 1981; Sheehy and Perkins 1976; Sooy et al 1973) have shown that the use of gelatin sponge (Gelfoam) as a seal for the oval window fenestra is associated with a high incidence of perilymph fistula. Sheehy and Perkins (1976) compared gelatin sponge fat and fascia as seals for the fenestra and found that the incidence of perilymph fistula was 3.5% when gelatin sponge was used, 1.9% when fat was used, and 0.6% when fascia was used. Lippy and Schuring (1984) compared the incidence of perilymph fistula formation with the use of gelatin sponge versus that of the Robinson vein graft prosthesis. They reported a significant difference: 50% for gelatin sponge and 4% for tissue seals. Gelatin sponge is found to be inadequate as an oval window seal because of the following reasons:

1. It may be resorbed before the neomembrane has formed.

2. The gelatin sponge will be softened by the perilymph, and the prosthesis will penetrate through the gelatin sponge, causing a perilymph fistula.

**3.** The neomembrane that forms with a gelatin sponge is very thin and is perforated repeatedly by the prosthesis, leading to the formation of a perilymph fistula.

Linthicum (1980) in his report provided evidence that gelatin sponge when used as an oval window seal is more likely to cause perilymph fistula. Causse and colleagues (1983) recommended using a tissue seal over the oval window fenestra to prevent perilymph fistula formation.

## LATE (DELAYED OR SECONDARY) PERILYMPH FISTULA

A late perilymph fistula can occur long after a successful stapedectomy. Morrison (1984) found that this is often the cause of sensorineural deafness that sometimes occurs long after a successful stapedectomy. Most authorities maintain that the longer stapedectomy patients are followed up, the greater the chances of perilymph fistula occurring. Morrison (1984) found that in 50% of late perilymph fistulae, no obvious cause could be discerned (in the other patients, mountaineering, lifting heavy objects, coughing, sneezing, pressure changes [barotrauma] from flying, and head injuries were suspected as the cause). Otitis media following stapedectomy is not likely to cause a perilymph fistula.

## HOW DOES A PERILYMPH FISTULA FORM?

Author Glasscock (1973) noted that the cochlear aqueduct is patent in a majority of adults. It puts the cerebrospinal fluid (CSF) in potential communication with the perilymph. Pressure in the CSF is transmitted directly to the perilymph. Shea (1974) noted that CSF pressure in the lumbar spine is 150 mm of water and that the pressure in the cistern through the cochlear aqueduct can be as high as 350 mm of water. In the event that the eustachian tube becomes blocked, negative pressure in the middle ear builds up and can reach −600 mm of water. Thus, a potential gradient of 950 mm of water is created, which can push the perilymph out of the vestibule. This can prevent the seal over the fenestra from healing, resulting in a perilymph fistula.

## CLINICAL FINDINGS

Clinical examination of the ear will appear normal to external appearances. Occasionally the tympanic membrane will be retracted.

## AUDIOMETRIC EVALUATION

Pure tone audiometry usually reveals sensorineural hearing loss in the low frequencies followed by a flat sensorineural hearing loss that fluctuates. Recruitment will be present in the initial stages, and short increment sensitivity index (SISI) scores are often above 75%. In the early stages, speech discrimination scores fluctuate with the pure tone thresholds; later on, they may lower disproportionately. A variable conductive hearing loss may be seen.

## VESTIBULAR TESTS

### Hallpike Caloric Tests

Canal paresis or a hypoactive response is a likely finding. It must be appreciated, however, that there is a high incidence of diminished caloric response. Thus, it becomes difficult to assess the true value of its significance in using it to diagnose the presence of a perilymph fistula.

### Electronystagmography

Electronystagmography (ENG) may reveal a direction fixed positional nystagmus, but, again, this cannot be used to diagnose a perilymph fistula.

### Fistula Test

Fistula tests with a pneumatic otoscope have been found to be negative in one third of the cases. Fistula tests with ENG, however, give a higher degree of accuracy. Beales (1981) reported that 16 patients who had a negative fistula test but in whom a fistula was suspected were reoperated to rule out a fistula. Only one had a perilymph fistula; out of six patients with a positive ENG fistula test, five were found to have a fistula. Thus, the incidence of false-positive and false-negative findings was low enough to make this test reasonably reliable.

## RADIOLOGICAL EVALUATION

Kosling et al (1995) reported on the use of high-resolution CT scanning to detect the presence of perilymph fistulae. They took high-resolution CT scans (1 mm slice thickness) in the axial and coronal planes The authors reported an air bubble (in the vestibule) at the end of the prosthesis to be an indirect sign of the presence of a perilymph fistula. This was the finding in six patients, and all six were found to have perilymph fistulae. Thus, CT scans were found to be of value in detecting the presence of perilymph fistulae poststapedectomy.

## HOW CAN A PERILYMPH FISTULA BE PREVENTED?

Intraoperatively, the surgeon should do the following:

1. Reflect the mucosa off the footplate completely before making a fenestra.
2. Perform stapedotomy technique, which is less likely to result in perilymph fistula formation.
3. Perform tissue graft seal over the fenestra, which acts as a barrier between the perilymph (vestibule) and the prosthesis (Fig. 12–2).
4. Place the prosthesis securely on the incus to prevent it from migrating.
5. Avoid using Gelfoam as a seal.

Postoperatively, the patient should do the following:

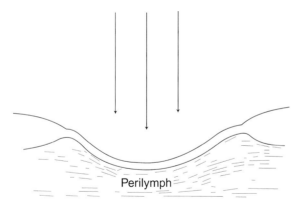

**Figure 12–2** A connective tissue seal prevents a peri-lymph fistula from forming. (*Adapted from Beales PH. Otosclerosis. Bristol: John Wright and Sons; 1981. Used with permission.*)

1. Avoid trauma to the head.

2. Cough and sneeze with the mouth wide open.

3. Avoid straining against a closed glottis.

4. Avoid the possibility of barotrauma for at least 1 month following stapedectomy.

5. Avoid lifting heavy weights.

6. Report immediately if symptoms such as vertigo, tinnitus, or hearing loss manifest themselves.

## MANAGEMENT OF A PERILYMPH FISTULA

Surgical closure of the fistula is the treatment of choice. Many surgeons consider this to be a surgical emergency. It is important that the field be kept dry to inspect the oval window area so as to see if perilymph oozes out. If the leak is not visible, then the patient's head should be lowered and the internal jugular vein on the same side compressed in an effort to make the leak visible.

Causse et al (1991) devised a test to help detect a perilymph fistula intraoperatively. They used a 1.0 mm diamond burr to remove fibrous adhesions from the oval window (this burr can now be replaced by lasers). To confirm that a fistula is present, they placed a small piece of Gelfoam at the site of the suspected fistula. They then tested it on Clinitest glucose test paper. If the paper turned red, perilymph fluid was present, indicating the presence of a perilymph fistula. Once the leak was detected, the fistulous tract was excised and the prosthesis removed.

Lasers have proven to be immensely helpful and are excellent working tools in managing perilymph fistulae. First, the mucosa over the footplate is elevated completely. Next, a fresh soft tissue seal is placed over an adequately created fenestra. A new adequate prosthesis is placed over the seal. The patient is advised total bed rest for 48 hours.

In a retrospective analysis of 26 cases, Pirodda et al (2002) reported on their findings of their approach to the management of rapid deterioration in bone conduction. Patients in their study had experienced deterioration in bone conduction some time after stapes surgery. Seven were treated conservatively with medication (i.e., pharmacologically), and the other 19 were treated with surgery and medication. Of the seven, improvement was seen in three, and in the other four, hearing remained unchanged. In the 19 cases managed with surgery and medication (in 5 cases, a perilymphatic fistula was found at surgical exploration), 4 cases improved, 4 worsened, and 11 experienced no change. The authors concluded their study by advocating an aggressive approach to the problem of perilymph fistulae.

## RESULTS OF TREATMENT OF PERILYMPH FISTULA

Improvement of hearing, especially once sensorineural hearing loss is present, is minimal because by then serous labyrinthitis has usually been well established. Early repair of perilymph fistulae does help symptoms such as vertigo resolve. Tinnitus may not resolve completely. Thus, the treatment of choice is to diagnose perilymph fistula early and to treat it as a surgical emergency.

## REFERENCES

Beales PH. The perilymph fistula after stapedectomy. In: *Otosclerosis.* Bristol: John Wright and Sons Ltd.; 1981:48–168.

Causse JB, Causse JR, Wiet RJ. Special conditions in otosclerosis surgery. In: Wiet RJ, Causse JB, Stambaugh GE, Causse JR, eds. *Otosclerosis (Otospongiosis).* American Academy of Otolaryngology—Head and Neck Surgery Foundation; Alexandria, Va; 1991:134–152.

Causse JB, Causse JR, Wiet RJ, Yoo TJ. Complications of stapedectomies. *Am J Otol.* 1983;4:275–280.

Crabtree JA, Britton BH, Powers WH. An evaluation of revision stapes surgery. *Laryngoscope.* 1980;90:224–227.

Derlacki EL. Revision stapes surgery: Problems with some solutions. *Laryngoscope.* 1985;95:1047–1053.

Feldman BA, Schuknecht HF. Experiences with revision stapedectomy procedures. *Laryngoscope.* 1970;80:1281–1291.

Glasscock ME. The stapes gusher. *Arch Otolaryngol.* 1973;98:82.

Glasscock ME, McKennan KX, Levine SC. Revision stapedectomy. *Otolaryngol— Head Neck Surg.* 1987;96:141–148.

Goodhill VH. The conductive hearing loss phenomenon in poststapedectomy perilymphatic fistulas. *Laryngoscope.* 1967;77:1179–1190.

Harrison WH, Shambaugh GE, Derlacki EL, Clemis JD. Perilymph fistula in stapes surgery. *Laryngoscope.* 1967;77:836–849.

Kosling S, Woldag K, Meister EF, Reschke I, Heywang-Kobrunner SH. Value of computed tomography in patients with persistent vertigo. *Invest Radiol.* 1995;30(12): 712–715.

Lewis ML. Inner ear complications of stapes surgery. *Laryngoscope.* 1961;71:377–383.

Linthicum FH. Histologic evidence of the causes of failure of in stapes surgery. *Ann Otol Rhinol Laryngol.* 1980;2:67–77.

Lippy WH, Schuring AG. Stapedectomy revision following sensorineural hearing loss. *Otolaryngol—Head Neck Surg.* 1984;92:580–582.

Matz GJ, Lockhart HB, Lindsay JR. Meningitis following stapedectomy. *Laryngoscope.* 1968;78:56–63.

Moon CN. Perilymph fistulas complicating the stapedectomy operation: A review of 49 cases. *Laryngoscope.* 1970;80:515–531.

Morrison AW. Otosclerosis diseases of the otic capsule. In: Ballantyne J, Groves J, eds. *Scott Brown's Diseases of the Ear, Nose and Throat.* Vol. 2. Boston: Butterworths; 1984:405–464.

Newlands WJ. Poststapedectomy otitis media and meningitis. *Arch Otolaryngol.* 1976;102(1):51–54.

Pirodda A, Modugno GC, Stamato R, Montaguti M, Ceroni AR. Late deterioration in bone conduction after stapes surgery: A retrospective analysis. *Acta Otorhinolaryngologica Italica.* 2002;22(3):119–126.

Shea JJ. Eversion of the lining of the membrane of the vestibule. *Laryngoscope.* 1974; 84:1122.

Sheehy JL, Nelson RA, House HP. Revision stapedectomy: A review of 258 cases. *Laryngoscope.* 1981;91:43–51.

Sheehy JL, Perkins JH. Stapedectomy: Gelfoam compared with tissue grafts. *Laryngoscope.* 1976;86:426–443.

Sooy FA, Owens E, Neufeld ES. Comparison of wire vein and wire Gelfoam prostheses in stapedectomy for otosclerosis. *Ann Otol, Rhinol Laryngol.* 1973;82:149–152.

Wiet RJ, Harvey SA, Bauer GP. Complications in stapes surgery: Options for prevention and management. *Otolaryngol Clin N Am.* 1993;26(3):471–490.

# Chapter *13*

# Sudden Sensorineural Hearing Loss Immediately Following Stapedectomy

One of the most dreaded complications following stapedectomy is sensorineural hearing loss, which may be partial or total. In general, the incidence varies from 0.6 to 3.0% (Hough 1966; Schuknecht 1962; Sheehy and House 1962).

Very frequently the exact cause is unknown, but one important cause of profound sensorineural deafness following stapedectomy is rupture of Reissner's membrane (Causse et al 1991). Reissner's membrane is a two-layered membrane that separates the endolymphatic space from the perilymphatic space. Excessive movement of the perilymph with increased perilymphatic pressure may rupture Reissner's membrane because the helicotrema constitutes too narrow a connection between the two spaces to achieve good compensation. A torn Reissner's membrane causes the cochlear action potentials to drop drastically, resulting in severe cochlear hearing loss.

## ETIOLOGY

### Serous Labyrinthitis

The exact causes of sensorineural hearing loss following stapedectomy are not known. It is thought, however, that serous labyrinthitis develops shortly after stapedectomy as part of the healing process that accompanies surgery (Wiet et al 1993). This type of labyrinthitis does resolve quickly. It may evoke symptoms such as mild gait unsteadiness, vertigo, and a slight decrease in hearing with reduced speech discrimination (Shea 1963). A decrease in hearing for frequencies above 2 kHz, along with reduced speech discrimination, is typical. The patient may also experience distortion, diplacusis, and recruitment. Symptoms usually resolve within a few days, although sometimes they may take several months to resolve (Shambaugh 1963). Patients who had preoperative endolymphatic hydrops may experience recrudescence of symptoms, especially if blood enters the vestibule (Wiet et al 1993). The ear that experiences serous labyrinthitis is more likely to go through the same experience at revision surgery. Serous labyrinthitis, however, usually resolves without sequelae. The temporary hearing loss that occurs in such situations must be distinguished from those that are permanent, irreversible, and progressive.

## Acoustic Trauma

Surgical trauma is the most prevalent. Schuknecht (1962) analyzed cases of profound sensorineural hearing loss following stapedectomy and reported that surgical trauma was the cause. Of these, 11 cases experienced profound sensorineural hearing loss as the result of extensive drilling. Other factors were traumatic mobilization of the stapes footplate, bleeding, and trauma with surgical instruments. If a microdrill has been used to create a fenestra on the footplate, it runs the risk of causing a sensorineural hearing loss. If a drill is to be used, it should have a higher torque and be used at a very slow speed in such a way that no vibrations are caused. The labyrinth is at risk if a fast rotation of the drill is carried out. It should also be observed that the ossicular chain should not be touched.

## Excessive Movement of the Stapes

Excessive movement of the stapes, especially if the footplate has not been fixed, can cause a hydraulic effect, which has the potential to damage the membranous structures of the vestibule.

## Inadvertent Rupture of the Membranous Inner Ear

The surgeon can inadvertently damage the membranous inner ear while trying to create a fenestra or while trying to retrieve bits of bone from the footplate that may have fallen into the vestibule. Such maneuvers are dangerous and should be discouraged.

## Rapid Loss of Perilymph

This can occur if the surgeon inadvertently applies a suction tip too close to the fenestra or if a perilymph gusher takes place. The surgeon must take care not to apply the suction near the fenestra. (Perilymph gushers, also known as CSF gushers, are discussed in Chapter 16.) Perilymph fistula is also a major cause of profound sensorineural hearing loss in the postoperative period; this is discussed in detail in Chapter 12.

A sudden release in perilymph pressure in patients who had some degree of endolymphatic hydrops preoperatively can result in sensorineural hearing loss. Postoperatively, this leads to tinnitus, vertigo, and a drop in all bone conduction thresholds. This progresses to profound sensorineural hearing loss that responds poorly to treatment. Causse (1980) recommended that any patient who presents with hydrops-like symptoms should avoid surgery and have symptoms properly under control for at least 6 months before undergoing surgery.

## Hydrops

Schuknecht (1962) reported on the basis of animal studies that hydrops was the most common reaction following stapedectomy and also the first to manifest itself in the postoperative period. He described five types of inner ear reactions to stapedectomy:

1. hydrops

2. hypotonic atrophy

**3.** acoustic trauma

**4.** serofibrinous labyrinthitis

**5.** suppurative labyrinthitis

Hypotonic atrophy is the likely result of fluid pressure imbalance and biochemical alterations of the cochlear fluids. Acoustic trauma presents as organ of Corti damage in the upper basal turn of the cochlea. Serofibrinous labyrinthitis occurs when the exudates are replaced by connective tissue. Suppurative labyrinthitis usually occurs secondary to infections in the middle ear. Associated findings in the study by Schuknecht (1962) were endolymphatic hydrops and advanced degeneration of the organ of Corti.

Causse (1980) in his personal series found that in 2% of cases, removal of too much of the bony rim at the annulus, subluxation of the incus, or increased negative pressure in the middle ear forced the prosthesis into the vestibule. This resulted in patients developing a pattern like Meniere's disease. Management consisted of steroids and early aeration of the middle ear.

The least common cause consisted of a sudden release of active enzymes from the otosclerotic focus into the inner ear. Causse (1980) believed that this leads to the destruction of the organ of Corti. Causse recommended that sodium fluoride therapy be introduced to help reduce the incidence of profound sensorineural hearing loss in such patients.

Numerous histopathologic specimens have demonstrated atrophy of the spiral ligament and stria vascularis in areas adjacent to endosteal involvement (Benitez and Schuknecht 1962; Hildyard et al 1972; Wiet et al 1987). Atrophy of the spiral ligament can lead to spontaneous rupture of the basilar membrane. The cochlea may be more vulnerable when involved with extensive otosclerosis with endosteal involvement and thus may be more susceptible to trauma induced by surgery. Those cases that have the most fragile cochlea usually have obliterative otosclerosis, which usually requires extensive drilling.

## TREATMENT

Careful monitoring of the patient's hearing in the immediate postoperative period is mandatory in order to detect those who are in danger of developing a profound irreversible hearing loss. If sensorineural hearing loss is indeed detected, repeated injections of intravenous nicotinic acid are given. This may be repeated four to five times a day. Intravenous heparin is given in small doses because of its vasodilator, antispasmodic actions. Hydrocortisone is also given.

## POSTOPERATIVE VERTIGO

Causse et al (1991) believed that the main cause of postoperative vertigo after stapedectomy is a change in pressure and excessive movement of the posterior labyrinthine fluids. The incidence of postoperative vertigo is reduced by avoiding excessive movement of the piston. Because transient hydrops is known to occur following stapedectomy, hydrops-reducing measures such as osmotic drugs and nicotinic acid have reduced the incidence, severity, and duration of vertigo following stapedectomy. It must be mentioned, however, that all patients who have vertigo at the time of a diagnosis of otosclerosis must have their symptoms under control for at least 6 months prior to surgery.

## TINNITUS IN THE POSTOPERATIVE PERIOD

Low- and medium-frequency tinnitus is related to the changes in pressure of the labyrinthine fluids. Even a minute change in labyrinthine fluid pressure is a biochemical stimulus for the outer hair cells of the organ of Corti. When there is no excessive fluid pressure, no action potential is discharged.

Tympanometry will demonstrate if the prosthesis is too short or has excessive penetration into the vestibule. Tinnitus is caused by excessive (rather than a lack of) penetration of the prosthesis into the vestibule. Although osmotic drugs may temporarily reduce tinnitus, only revision surgery can produce permanent improvement (Causse et al 1991). Tinnitus present prior to surgery is considered to be of vascular or enzymatic origin and is thought to be related to the natural progress of the otosclerotic disease. Sodium fluoride should be given to such patients prior to surgery because it is found to reduce the intensity of the tinnitus.

## REFERENCES

Benitez JT, Schuknecht HF. Otosclerosis: A human temporal bone report. *Laryngoscope.* 1962;72:1–9.

Causse JB. Etiology and therapy of cochlear hydrops following stapedectomy. *Am J Otolaryngol.* 1980;1:221–224.

Causse JB, Causse JR, Wiet RJ. Complications in stapes surgery. In: Wiet RJ, Causse JB, Shambaugh GE, Causse JR, eds. *Otosclerosis (Otospongiosis).* American Academy of Otolaryngology—Head and Neck Surgery Foundation; Alexandria, Va; 1991:153–162.

Hildyard VH, Sando I, Davison SL. Diagnosis and management of far advanced otosclerosis. *Arch Otolaryngol.* 1972;96:530–534.

Hough JVD. Recent advances in otosclerosis. *Arch Otolaryngol.* 1972;83:379–390.

Schuknecht HF. Sensorineural hearing loss following stapedectomy. *Arch Otolaryngol.* 1962;54:336–347.

Shambaugh GE. Cochlear pathology after stapes surgery. *Arch Otolaryngol.* 1963;78: 214–219.

Shea JL. Complications of the stapedectomy operation. *Ann Otol, Rhinol, Laryngol.* 1963;72:1109–1123.

Sheehy JL, House HP. Causes of failure in stapes surgery. *Laryngoscope.* 1962;73: 10–31.

Wiet RJ, Harvey SA, Bauer GP. Complications in stapes surgery. *Otolaryngol Clin N Am.* 1993;26(3):471–490.

Wiet RJ, Morgenstein SA, Zwolan TA, Pircon SM. Far advanced otosclerosis. *Arch of Otolaryngol—Head Neck Surg.* 1987;113:299–302.

# Chapter *14*

## Stapedectomy versus Stapedotomy

Stapedectomy has evolved from total removal of the footplate to the small fenestra technique. Improvement of hearing, especially improvement of speech discrimination scores, has been cited as justification for employing the small fenestra technique for most stapedectomies. Studies on the small fenestra technique suffer from design flaws, however, creating a bias in favor of the technique (Rizer and Lippy 1993). Variables such as type of prosthesis and oval window seal were not considered.

### REVIEW OF THE LITERATURE

Smyth and Hassard (1978) reviewed 800 stapedectomies, examining the incidence of complications and their relationship with the size of the fenestra created. They reported that, in terms of hearing, the small fenestra technique and the total footplate removal were virtually the same. They found, however, that the small fenestra technique had fewer complications such as perilymph fistula and delayed sensorineural hearing loss.

McGee (1981) analyzed 280 stapedectomies and correlated the relationship between fenestra size and improvement of hearing. He reported an improvement in hearing with the small fenestra technique, although his study had many variables, such as different prostheses used for the procedures, different oval window seals, and the amount of footplate removed.

Shea (1982) reported better high-frequency hearing and a lower incidence of complications with the small fenestra technique. Moon and Hahn (1984), on the other hand, reported that in their series, although small fenestra stapedectomy improved hearing in the high frequencies, the results did not warrant a change in technique.

In their report on hearing results in otosclerosis surgery, Persson et al (1997) compared the findings in patients who had undergone partial stapedectomy, total stapedectomy, and stapedotomy. They examined the hearing results in a consecutive series of 407 patients with otosclerosis who had undergone primary stapes surgery. In all, there were 437 ears that were operated on. Partial stapedectomy was performed on 70 ears (16%), and total stapedectomy was performed on 205 ears (47%). In both groups the House steel wire prosthesis on fascia was used. The remaining 162 ears (37%) had a stapedotomy performed using the Fisch 0.4 mm Teflon platinum piston. Persson et al reported that none of these patients in this series presented with sensorineural hearing loss (> 15 dB). The comparison between the three groups 1 year postoperatively showed that the air-bone gap was smaller for partial and total stapedectomy than for stapedotomy for all frequencies except at 4 kHz. The air-bone gap was calculated as the difference between the preoperative bone conduction and the postoperative air conduction thresholds. Partial and total stapedectomy also showed larger improvements of bone conduction thresholds compared with stapedotomy for all frequencies except 4 kHz. At the 3-year follow-up, the hearing gain for all frequencies (250 Hz to 8 kHz) was larger for partial and total stapedectomy as compared with stapedotomy. Yet when comparing the decline of hearing from 1 to 3 years postoperatively, the hearing gain achieved with partial and total stapedectomy was much more rapid than with stapedotomy. These results showed that, in the short term, partial or total stapedectomy gives better hearing results even at high frequencies. Stapedotomy, on the other hand, yielded more stable hearing results over time. Persson et al (1997) concluded that, all things considered, good stable hearing results as seen with stapedotomy were preferable to a good initial result, which was likely to deteriorate over time, as seen with partial and total stapedectomy.

Spandow et al (2000) conducted a retrospective study where they analyzed the results of 60 stapedectomies with the Schuknecht method, and 55 stapedotomies with the Fisch method. The hearing benefit was maximum 1 year after surgery for both procedures. The improvement of the air conduction thresholds, however, was greater in the stapedotomy procedure than in the stapedectomy group. Both groups maintained significantly improved hearing over a period of 10 years (although thresholds became worse gradually over a period of time). There was just one "dead ear" and two ruptured chorda tympani in the stapedectomy group but none in the stapedotomy group. The authors concluded that stapedotomy with the Fisch-type prosthesis is a safe procedure when performed by an experienced surgeon.

## RATIONALE FOR USING THE SMALL FENESTRA TECHNIQUE

Marquet et al (1972) described the surface tension of perilymph to be an important factor in the protection of the labyrinth during surgery upon the footplate. Following stapedectomy, the surface tension of the perilymph, together with the contact angle of the perilymph on the prosthesis, determines the shape of the reparative soft tissue that will close the fenestra. The concave shape of the meniscus protects the labyrinth by preventing footplate particles from entering the vestibule. In a small fenestra footplate, particles are very minimal and are less traumatic. This procedure produces complete closure of the air-bone gap in the high frequencies.

The middle ear is an impedance matching device that changes sound energy into mechanical energy. In stapedectomy, the prosthesis attempts to simulate the action of the footplate and the annular ligament complex. Causse et al (1993) suggested that a small fenestra in the footplate provides adequate energy in the tip of the piston but does not provide adequate energy in more distal portions of the cochlea. Consequently, the high-pitched tones in the basal part of the cochlea give successful hearing results from stapedotomy. However, mid- and low-frequency tones in the apical portion of the cochlea give less successful hearing results because the energy does not reach the apical cochlea adequately. Total stapedectomy can give successful results at the mid and low frequencies but less successful results in the high frequencies.

Causse et al (1993) reported that the annular ligament of the stapes footplate has significant elastic fibers that add resistance as a mode of protection from excessive vibration. Vein grafts have more elastic fibers 2 years after being transplanted into the middle ear when compared with their initial harvest from the arm. The prosthesis and the vein graft act as a single unit, mechanically stimulating the vestibule. The vein graft acts as a trampoline where distortion of the undersurface of the trampoline is not related to small changes in the width of the vibrating body (diameter of the prosthesis), especially if the size of the vibrating body is small compared with the overall surface of the trampoline (fenestra). The vein dampens or attenuates the effect of the prosthesis on the basal turn so that no hearing ability is lost. If the fenestra is too small and the vein graft too thick, the acoustic impedance changes, and an inadequate amount of energy is transmitted to the apical cochlea, affecting mid- and low-frequency tones.

Causse et al (1991) provided additional reasons for using the small fenestra technique. The fenestra should be approximately 0.8 mm and should be placed in the posterior half of the footplate. Their rationale is the following:

1. The utricle and saccule are located under the anterior two thirds of the footplate and thus will not be traumatized by the prosthesis.

2. A small fenestra avoids the release of proteolytic enzymes into the labyrinth by rupture of the otosclerotic focus, which is located anteriorly.

3. The small fenestra technique procedure avoids any rupture of neovessels in the otosclerotic focus.

4. This procedure allows reconstitution of good impedance and compliance around the piston. If the portion of the vein graft located between the rim of the footplate fenestra and the piston edge is approximately 0.2 mm in size, there will be sufficient anatomophysiologic reconstitution of a pseudoannular ligament. The small fenestra technique behaves in the same manner as the annular ligament would. Explained simply, the seal over the small fenestra acts as a trampoline, exerting pressure equally in all directions. Furthermore, the labyrinth would not be traumatized in this situation.

## WHAT ARE THE RECOMMENDED DIMENSIONS OF THE SMALL FENESTRA?

Most reports recommend a dimension of 0.6 to 0.8 mm (Dubreuil et al 1994).

## WHERE SHOULD THE FENESTRA BE PLACED?

The fenestra should be placed in the posterior half of the footplate in order to avoid trauma to the saccule.

## WHAT IS THE INSTRUMENT OF CHOICE FOR CREATING THE FENESTRA?

Most reports favor using a laser to create the small fenestra. The authors generally cite precision as the prime reason for using the laser. Other advantages are an established safety profile and few complications when a laser is used. There are some reports, however, that cite the equally safe use of a microdrill to create a small fenestra (Sedwick et al 1997).

## WHICH PROSTHESIS SHOULD BE USED FOR A STAPEDOTOMY?

The piston-type prosthesis should be used; stapedotomy permits the use of a piston-type prosthesis only.

## ADVANTAGES AND DISADVANTAGES OF STAPEDECTOMY

The advantages of stapedectomy include the following:

1. Relatively easier to perform
2. Good closure of the air-bone gap (Kos et al 2001)

The disadvantages include the following:

1. Relatively more traumatic to the inner ear
2. Decline in hearing results over time.
3. Relatively more complications such as sensorineural hearing loss

## ADVANTAGES AND DISADVANTAGES OF STAPEDOTOMY

The advantages of stapedotomy include the following: (Laitakari and Laitakari 1997):

1. Less traumatic to the inner ear
2. Stable hearing results over time (Levy et al 1990)
3. Fewer complications such as perilymph fistula (Kursten et al 1994)

The disadvantages include the following:

1. Technically more difficult to perform

**2.** Closure of air-bone gap not as good as with partial stapedectomy

## CHOOSING BETWEEN STAPEDECTOMY (PARTIAL OR TOTAL) AND STAPEDOTOMY

The surgeon should employ the technique that consistently and reliably brings about the best possible results. The results should be able to withstand the tests of time and should be stable. Should the surgeon start out to perform a small fenestra stapedotomy but is unable to do so, he should then settle for a safe, atraumatic, and reliable procedure as the circumstances demand. The operating surgeon should be flexible enough to adapt to the needs of the situation rather than be a slave to one particular technique.

At all times, the procedure should be done in as atraumatic a manner as possible, with correct positioning of the prosthesis.

## COMMENTS

Small fenestra stapedotomy has been reported in the literature as an improvement over total stapedectomy. Rizer and Lippy (1993), however, believed that this indicates a bias rather than a real improvement in technique. Their findings reveal that moderate removal of the footplate provides good results. They found that

**1.** A small fenestra cannot be achieved in all cases.

**2.** Overclosure is less common with stapedotomy than with total stapedectomy.

**3.** All techniques—small fenestra stapedotomy and partial and total stapedectomies—achieve the same hearing result at 4 kHz.

## NEW DEVELOPMENTS

Stapedioplasty is a new technique being advocated by Poe (2000). Using a laser, Poe vaporized the anterior crus and mobilized the posterior portion of the footplate. This eliminated the need for a stapedial prosthesis. This technique, however, is useful only when the otosclerotic focus is limited to the anterior portion of the footplate. Similarly, Silverstein and colleagues (2002) reported on laser stapedotomy minus prosthesis (laser STAMP). This is in essence the same technique as described by Poe (2000). Silverstein et al in particular looked at refixation of the newly mobilized footplate. They concluded that laser STAMP is a minimally invasive procedure that, over the follow-up period, has a very low incidence of refixation, as evidenced by a lack of progressive conductive hearing loss. The success of this procedure depends on the correct selection of patients. Only those patients who have an otosclerotic focus limited to the anterior portion of the footplate are considered suitable candidates for this procedure. Silverstein et al found that laser STAMP is a viable alternative to conventional stapedotomy, yielding good results without evidence of refixation of the footplate.

## SUMMARY

Small fenestra stapedotomy provides better hearing results, especially in the high-frequency range, and is associated with fewer complications. Equally important as the creation of the small fenestra is atraumatic technique, a good seal using connective tissue rather than Gelfoam, and a good prosthesis.

Rizer and Lippy (1993) noted that the literature shows a bias in favor of small fenestra stapedotomy over total stapedectomy. They report equally good results in partial footplate removal stapedectomy with no complications.

Laser STAMP seems to offer a valuable alternative to conventional stapedotomy, even though its application is limited to patients who have an otosclerosis focus limited to the anterior portion of the footplate.

## REFERENCES

Causse JB, Causse JR, Wiet RJ. Surgical treatment. In: Wiet RJ, Causse JB, Shambaugh GE, Causse JR, eds. *Otosclerosis (Otospongiosis).* American Academy of Otolaryngology—Head and Neck Surgery; Alexandria, Va; 1991:107–126.

Causse JB, Gherini S, Lopez A, Juberthie L, Oliver JC, Bastianelli G. Impedance transfer: Acoustic impedance of the annular ligament and stapedial tendon reconstruction in otosclerosis surgery. *Am J Otolaryngol.* 1993;14:613–617.

Dubreuil C, Bouchayer M, Boulud B, Di Brango P, Reiss T. Otosclerosis: Stapedectomy or stapedotomy: A long term comparative study. *Annales d'Otolaryngologie et de chirurgie cervici faciale.* 1994;111(5):249–264.

Kos MI, Montandon PB, Guyot JP. Short and long term results of stapedotomy and stapedectomy with a Teflon wire piston prosthesis. *Ann Otol, Rhinol Laryngol.* 2001;110(10):907–911.

Kursten R, Schneider B, Zrunek M. Long term results after stapedectomy versus stapedotomy. *Am J Otolaryngol.* 1994;15(6):804–806.

Laitakari K, Laitakari E. From posterior crus stapedectomy to 0.6 mm stapedotomy: towards reliability in otosclerosis surgery. *Acta Otolaryngol.* 1997;529(suppl): 50–52.

Levy R, Shvero J, Hadar T. Stapedotomy technique and results: Ten years' experience and comparative study. *Laryngoscope.* 1990;100(10, pt 1):1097–1099.

Marquet J, Creten WC, Van Camp KI. Consideration about the surgical approach in stapedectomy. *Acta Otolaryngol.* 1972;74:406–411.

McGee TM. Comparison of small fenestra and total stapedectomy *Ann Otol Rhinol Laryngol.* 1981;90:630–632.

Moon CN, Hahn MJ. Partial versus total footplate removal in stapedectomy: A comparative study. *Laryngoscope.* 1984;94:912–915.

Persson P, Harder H, Magnuson B. Hearing results in otosclerosis surgery after partial stapedectomy, total stapedectomy, and stapedotomy. *Acta Otolaryngol.* 1997; 117(1):94–99.

Poe DS. Laser assisted endoscopic stapedectomy: A prospective study. *Laryngoscope.* 2000;110(5, pt 2, suppl 95):1–37.

Rizer FM, Lippy WH. Evolution of techniques of stapedectomy from total stapedectomy to small fenestra stapedectomy. *Otolaryngol Clin N Am.* 1993; 26:443–451.

Sedwick JD, Louden CL, Shelton C. Stapedectomy vs. stapedotomy: Do you really need a laser? *Arch Otolaryngol—Head Neck Surg.* 1997;123(2):177–180.

Shea JJ. Stapedectomy: A long term report. *Ann Otol, Rhinol Laryngol.* 1982;91: 516–520.

Silverstein H, Jackson LE, Conlon WS, Rosenberg SI, Thompson JH. Laser stapedo-tomy minus prosthesis (laser STAMP): Absence of refixation. *Otol Neurotol.* 2002; 23(2):152–157.

Smyth GD, Hassard TH. Eighteen years' experience in stapedectomy: The case for the small fenestra operation. *Ann Otol Rhinol Laryngol.* 1978;49(suppl):3–36.

Spandow O, Soderberg O, Lennart B. Long term results in otosclerotic patients oper-ated on by stapedectomy or stapedotomy. *Scand Audiol.* 2000;29:186–190.

# Chapter 15

# Bilateral Otosclerosis and Revision Stapedectomy

Whether otosclerosis is unilateral or bilateral, the medical treatment is the same. The question that confronts otosclerosis surgeons is, rather, should both ears undergo stapedectomy? This is a controversial subject, with many experts for and others against (Porter et al 1995; Smyth et al 1975). It has been found that even with the best techniques, permanent cochlear hydrops can result from surgery on the second ear. Causse et al (1991) found that about one patient in 7000 develops profound sensorineural hearing loss.

## RECOMMENDED INTERVAL OF TIME BETWEEN SURGERIES

Causse et al (1991) recommended that the second ear be operated on after a minimum period of 1 year only if the other ear is doing well in terms of hearing and vestibular symptoms. They reasoned that surgically induced severe cochlear deterioration usually occurs within the first year postoperatively. If any problem occurs after that time, it usually manifests itself as a conductive hearing loss.

## CONTRAINDICATIONS FOR SECOND EAR STAPEDECTOMY

The two main contraindications for second ear stapedectomy are the following:

1. If the patient develops complications following the first surgery, then the second ear should not be operated on.
2. If the patient develops tinnitus and/or persistent vertigo following surgery upon the first ear, then stapedectomy should not be carried out on the second ear.

## ARGUMENTS AGAINST SECOND EAR STAPEDECTOMY

The main arguments against second ear stapedectomy can be summarized in this way:

1. It is impossible to guarantee a long-term successful result.

2. The second ear should be preserved in the event that the operated ear deteriorates.

3. The actual figures reported of sensorineural hearing loss may be higher than those reported because many patients are lost to follow-up.

4. An initial successful stapedectomy can fail many years later, resulting in profound sensorineural deafness.

5. Today there is a marked decrease in the number of patients undergoing stapedectomy, leaving younger surgeons with less experience in dealing with these complicated and technically challenging problems.

6. An inexperienced surgeon should never operate on the second ear.

## FACTORS THAT INFLUENCE THE SUCCESSFUL OUTCOME OF SECOND EAR STAPEDECOTMY

Middle ear abnormalities, which are quite common, can adversely affect the success of stapedectomy (Daniels et al 2001). Very reasonable rates of success, however, can be achieved even in the presence of bilateral middle ear abnormalities.

In prognosticating success to patients who are to undergo surgery on the second ear, the surgeon should consider the following:

1. If the first ear was anatomically normal and the procedure was successful, there is a 95% chance that the procedure in the second ear will be successful too (Daniels et al 2001).

2. Most abnormalities occur at a bilateral rate of approximately 25% in the other ear. However, the incidence of bilateral obliterated footplate is 41%, and the bilateral success rate is approximately 60%.

3. The other abnormalities with reduced rates of bilateral success include promontory overhang, malleus fixation, and a dehiscent or overhanging facial nerve.

Abnormal middle ear findings during stapedectomy occur in a significant percentage of patients. Reasonable rates of success and overclosure can still be expected, but this is findings-specific. Understanding this, the percentage of bilateral abnormalities and its impact on predicting rates of success can help the surgeon counsel the patient correctly.

It should not be the patient's request for second ear surgery that directs the surgeon regarding his or her decision to perform such surgery. Instead, it should be the surgeon's opinion regarding the patient's general and otological health that should dictate his or her decision.

With this goal in mind, the surgeon should be familiar with all the nuances of stapedectomy, should be very experienced, and should have the best possible equipment for performing the surgery.

## REVISION STAPEDECTOMY

Horn et al (1998) stated that revision stapedectomy offers neither the safety nor the success that is usually associated with primary stapes surgery. The increased surgical variables encountered during revision stapedectomy adversely affect the outcome, resulting in overall decreased air-bone gap closure to approximately 50% and sensorineural hearing loss greater than 1% in most series where mechanical (i.e., where a laser has not been used) revision of primary stapes has been undertaken.

Histopathologic studies in stapedectomy patients conducted by Hohmann (1962), Linthicum (1971), and Schuknecht (1974) have shown adhesions between the prosthesis or the oval window neomembrane and the utricle and saccule. Surgical manipulation of the prosthesis or neomembrane could rupture these delicate inner ear structures, resulting in permanent profound sensorineural hearing loss accompanied by vertigo. Yet the surgeon must uncover the reason why a stapedectomy has failed; this will entail manipulating the various structures in the middle ear and running the risk of a permanent sensorineural hearing loss.

The introduction of lasers for revision stapedectomy has significantly contributed to improvement in hearing while lessening the incidence of complications. Argon, KTP, and carbon dioxide lasers have all been reported to be very useful in revision stapedectomy (Lesinski and Stein 1989; McGee et al 1993; Palva and Ramsey 1990).

## CAUSES OF THE REAPPEARANCE OF A CONDUCTIVE HEARING LOSS FOLLOWING STAPEDECTOMY

Most authors (Ayache et al 2000; Fisch et al 2001) report that the most common causes for residual conductive hearing loss or the reappearance of a conductive hearing loss following stapedectomy include migration (displacement) of the stapes prosthesis, erosion of the incus, and bony or fibrous growth of the otosclerotic focus at the oval window. Ayache et al retrospectively reviewed a series of 26 revision stapedectomies. The leading cause of reappearance of a conductive hearing loss was prosthesis malfunction (migration) (42%), fibrous adhesions (37.5%), incus erosion (12.5%), and regrowth of the otosclerotic focus (12.5%). When revision was indicated because of cochleovestibular symptoms, middle ear exploration revealed three problems: oval window granuloma, excessively long prosthesis, and perilymph fistula.

Nadol (2001) reviewed the cases of 22 patients who had had stapedectomy for otosclerosis who then went on to develop a conductive hearing loss (CHL) of 10 dB or greater (air-bone gap averaged at 500 Hz and 1, 2, 3, and 4 kHz using postoperative air and bone conduction levels). The most common cause of CHL following stapedectomy was resorptive osteitis of the incus at the site of prosthesis attachment (64%), obliteration of the round window by otosclerosis (23%), the presence of the prosthesis lying on a fragment of stapedial footplate (23%) or abutting the bony margin of the oval window rather than centered on the fenestra (18%), and the presence of postoperative new bone formation in the oval window (14%).

## Incus Erosion (Resorptive Osteitis)

In his commentary on the findings seen at histopathology, Nadol (2001) noted that in situations where resorptive osteitis (RO) was suspected as the cause of CHL following stapedectomy, RO was seen as an exclusive finding in only 1 of 14 cases. In the remaining 13 cases where RO was thought to be the leading cause, other findings were noticed. They included round window obliteration, residual footplate fragment underlying the prosthesis, the prosthesis abutting the margin of the oval window, perilymph fistula, subluxation of the malleoincudal joint, new bone formation in the oval window, fibrocystic degeneration, and a dense fibrous plug in the oval window.

The causes of RO of the incus are thought to be pressure necrosis, medial fixation of the strut (Morgenstein and Manace 1968), a loose crimp, and damage to the mucosa enveloping the incus, which is presumed to provide anastamotic blood supply to the incus (Alberti 1965; Anson et al 1964). Gibbin (1979) noted that other middle ear pathologies attributable to stapes surgery included fibrosis and adhesions in the middle ear, intratympanic granuloma, and retraction of the tympanic membrane onto the incus. All these pathologies point to a postoperative inflammation as a common etiology.

In a series by Lesinski (1998), partial incus erosion on the undersurface of the incus was observed in 58% of cases and complete erosion in an additional 30% of cases. Lesinski notes that the longer the delay between the onset of the conductive hearing loss and the repair and revision, the greater the degree of incus erosion.

Partial incus erosion (less than 50%) can usually be repaired with a standard Lippy-Robinson bucket handle prosthesis. If the long process extends more than 1 mm below the facial ridge, a Robinson-Moon-Lippy stainless steel prosthesis with offset shaft produces consistent results. If the long process of the incus is too short, then a malleus to footplate prosthesis is used. McElveen (1998) used bone cement (Oto-Cement) to reconstruct the long process of the incus.

Lesinski (1998) noted that incus erosion (RO) was usually the result of biological bone vibrating against a fixed inert prosthesis. A loosely crimped wire loop prosthesis was usually the cause of incus erosion. Overcrimping was never a factor. The erosion invariably began on the undersurface of the incus, and the longer the duration of the conductive hearing loss, the greater the degree of erosion. Early revision of stapedectomy is usually associated with prosthesis migration (75% of cases in Lesinski's series) and a minimal degree of erosion of the incus. Hearing results with revision stapedectomy are improved when the prosthesis can be attached to the incus rather than attached directly from the malleus to the oval window.

Nadol (2001) postulated that RO of the incus could be caused by the differential motion of the incus at the junction of its attachment to the prosthesis. Thus, if motion of the prosthesis is limited by fibrosis, for example, this would in turn lead to movement of the attachment portion of the prosthesis with reference to the incus. This leads to friction between the prosthesis and the incus, which could result in resorptive osteitis.

## Obliteration of the Round Window by Otosclerosis

Nadol (2001) commented that, in his series, the incidence was high (5 out of 22 cases) and noted that in the literature such a finding is uncommon. He stated that in the operative notes, the operating surgeon had neglected to mention the condition of the status of the round window. Nadol therefore advocated that all otosclerosis surgeons carefully inspect the round window and check for its patency at the time of primary stapedectomy. If round window obliteration by otosclerosis is present, then it should be dealt with during the primary surgery. This would help reduce unnecessary revision procedures.

## Prosthesis Abutting the Bony Margin of the Oval Window or on Residual Footplate Fragments

This finding was observed in 9 of 22 cases reviewed by Nadol (2001). To prevent this from occurring, Nadol advocated excellent and meticulous technique. Blood can obscure complete visualization of the footplate, which in turn can lead to the creation of an inadequate fenestra, which can cause the prosthesis to migrate to the fragments, resulting in a postoperative conductive hearing loss. Excellent hemostasis and proper magnification can help visualize the footplate. Additionally, creation of a clean and adequate fenestra will minimize the chance of such an event from occurring.

## Malleus Fixation

This finding is low in the review by Nadol (2001). However, malleus fixation should be recognized as far as possible in the preoperative period; this is discussed in detail in Chapter 16. Briefly, it may be stated here that with the pneumatic otoscope it is possible to determine if malleus fixation is present. If the excursion of the tympanic membrane is shallow during the inflation of the bulb, then malleus fixation is more likely to be present. Intraoperatively, the surgeon must check the mobility of each individual ossicle independently. When malleus fixation is detected, it has to be dealt with in the appropriate manner.

## New Bone Formation in the Oval Window

In the series by Nadol (2001), new bone formation occurred when a drill-out technique for oval window obliteration was used. Nadol noted that the new bone appeared to be consistent with reparative rather than otosclerotic bone. This was seen exclusively in those patients who required a drill-out for an obliterated oval window. Lindsay (1961) reported similar findings when new bone formation occurred after an obliterated oval window required a drill-out. The clinical implication of this finding is that when a drill is used to drill out an extensively obliterated oval window, the surgeon should expect the formation of new bone. Thus, the surgeon should make the final fenestra much larger than the piston prosthesis to accommodate the occurrence of new bone formation without its resulting in a postoperative conductive hearing loss. Nadol concluded his report by stating that there are other etiologies at work that could cause a conductive hearing loss, notably piston diameter.

A piston diameter of 0.8 mm is adequate. A piston diameter of 0.3 mm, however, could result in a conductive hearing loss.

## INSTRUMENT OF CHOICE FOR REVISION STAPEDECTOMY

The laser is the instrument of choice for revision stapedectomy (Horn et al 1998; Lesinski 1998; Vernick and Kartush 1998).

## CRITERIA FOR REVISION STAPEDECTOMY

The criteria for revision stapedectomy include the following:

1. Revision stapes surgery is generally reserved for patients who continue to have a conductive hearing loss after initial hearing improvement.

2. Progressive, fluctuating sensorineural hearing loss or incapacitating vertigo will need exploration. A perilymphatic fistula should be expected.

3. Because revision stapes surgery does not yield the same results, a larger air-bone gap is needed as an indication for surgery. In the experience of Horn et al (1994), more than 90% of their revision stapes surgeries have a closure to 20 dB or less; therefore, they use a 20 dB air-bone gap as a minimum for revision surgery.

## RESULTS OF REVISION STAPEDECTOMY

Crabtree et al (1980) reported on 35 cases that were revised without the use of a laser. Forty-six percent of these cases achieved closure to within 10 dB, and 20% resulted in worse hearing or a dead ear. Sheehy et al (1981) reported on 258 other cases that were revised without the use of a laser; 44% achieved closure to within 10 dB, and only 7% had worse hearing or a dead ear. Lippy et al (1980) revised 100 cases without a laser and achieved closure to within 10 dB in 71% of cases, with 3.3% resulting in worse hearing or a dead ear.

Lesinski and Stein (1989) revised 59 cases with a carbon dioxide laser and achieved closure to within 10 dB in 66% of cases, with only 3% of patients experiencing worse hearing or a dead ear. Palva and Ramsey (1990) revised 82 cases using the argon laser and achieved closure to within 10 dB in 75% of cases, with only 3.5% resulting in worse hearing or a dead ear following the revision. McGee et al (1993) revised 77 cases and achieved closure to within 10 dB in 80.5% of cases, with 3.9% of patients experiencing worse hearing or a dead ear.

## RECOMMENDATIONS

Among the recommendations for revision stapedectomy are the following:

1. An experienced otosclerosis surgeon should perform a revision stapedectomy.

2. A laser should be used when performing a revision stapedectomy.

3. Revision stapedectomy should be performed at the earliest time. Attaching the prosthesis to the incus has a better chance of improving hearing. Some authors (e.g., Lippy 1994) recommend waiting for 6 weeks after the primary surgery before revising the stapedectomy to allow the postoperative reaction to resolve; otherwise bleeding and edema will impede surgery.

4. Local anesthesia should be used when operating on a revision in order to better monitor vertigo and hearing losses.

5. A tissue seal should be used over the oval window. If fistulae of the oval window are present, they may not always be evident. A tissue seal will close even those fistulae that are not apparent. The tissue seal produced by absorbable gelatin sponge will not safely support a rigid piston.

6. There is controversy as to whether the neomembrane interfacing between the prosthesis and the vestibule should be opened. In cases of doubt or difficulty, the neomembrane should be left alone. If the neomembrane is manipulated blindly, a profound sensorineural hearing loss could result.

7. When otosclerosis regrowth is encountered, the growth should be left alone. The hearing gain is temporary in such patients because the bone will regrow again, impeding hearing.

8. If the problem cannot be identified (i.e., there are negative findings), those cases with the tissue seal should be left undisturbed.

## REFERENCES

Alberti PWRM. The blood supply of the long process of the incus and the head of the stapes. *J Laryngol Otol.* 1965;79:964–970.

Anson BJ, Harper DC, Winch TR. Intraosseous blood supply of the auditory ossicles in man. *Ann Otol, Rhinol Laryngol.* 1964;73:645–658.

Ayache D, El Kihel M, Betsch C, Bou Malhab F, Elbaz P. Revision surgery of otosclerosis: A review of 26 cases. *Annales d'Oto-laryngologie et de Chirurgie Cervico Faciale.* 2000;117(5):281–290.

Causse JB, Causse JR, Wiet RJ. Special conditions in otosclerosis surgery. In: Wiet RJ, Causse JB, Shambaugh GE, Causse JR, eds. *Otosclerosis (Otospongiosis).* American Academy of Otolaryngology—Head and Neck Surgery Foundation; 1991:134–152.

Crabtree JA, Britton BH, Powers WH. An evaluation of revision stapes surgery. *Laryngoscope.* 1980;90:224–227.

Daniels RL, Krieger LW, Lippy WH. The other ear: findings and results in 1,800 bilateral stapedectomies. *Otol Neurotol.* 2001;22:603–607.

Fisch U, Acar GO, Huber AM. Malleostapedotomy in revision surgery for otosclerosis. *Otol Neurotol.* 2001;22(6):776–785.

Gibbin KP (1979): The histopathology of the incus after stapedectomy. *Clin Otolaryngol.* 1979;4:343–354.

Hohmann A. Inner ear reactions to stapes surgery (animal experiments). In: Schuknecht F, ed. *Otosclerosis.* Boston: Harvard University Press; 1962:305–317.

Horn KL, Gherini SG, Franz DC. Argon laser revision stapedectomy. *Am J Otol.* 1994;15:383–388.

Horn KL, Gherini SG, Griffin GM. Revision stapes surgery using the fiberoptic argon laser. *Oper Tech Otolaryngol—Head Neck Surg.* 1998;9(2)88–93.

Lesinski SG. Revision surgery for otosclerosis: 1998 perspective. *Oper Tech Otolaryngol—Head Neck Surg.* 1998;9(2):72–82.

Lesinski SG, Stein JA. Stapedectomy revision with CO2 laser. *Laryngoscope.* 1989;99:13–19.

Lindsay JR. Histologic findings following stapedectomy and polyethylene tube inserts in the human. *Ann Otol.* 1961;70:785–807.

Linthicum F. Histologic evidence of the cause of failure in stapes surgery. *Ann Otol, Rhinol Laryngol.* 1971;80:67–77.

Lippy WH. Special problems of otosclerosis surgery. In: Brackmann DE, Shelton CS, Arraiaga M, eds. *Otologic Surgery.* Philadelphia: WB Saunders; 1994:348–355.

Lippy WH, Schuring AG, Ziv M. Stapedectomy revision. *Am J Otol.* 1980;2:15–21.

McElveen JT. Repair of incus erosion with bone cement. *Oper Tech Otolaryngol—Head Neck Surg.* 1998;9(2):94–97.

McGee TM, Diaz Ordaz EA, Kartush JM. The role of KTP laser in revision stapedectomy. *Otolaryngol Head Neck Surg.* 1993;109:839–843.

Morgenstein KM, Manace ED. Incus necrosis following stapedectomy. *Laryngoscope.* 1968;78:600–619.

Nadol JB. Histopathology of residual and recurrent conductive hearing loss after stapedectomy. *Otol Neurotol.* 2001;22:162–169.

Palva T, Ramsey H. Revision surgery for otosclerosis. *Acta Otolaryngol.* 1990;110:416–420.

Porter MJ, Zeitoun H, Brookes GB. The Glasgow benefit plot used to assess the effect of bilateral stapedectomy. *Clin Otolaryngol.* 1995;20:68–71.

Schuknecht H. *Pathology of the Ear.* Cambridge, MA: Harvard University Press; 1974.

Sheehy JL, Nelson RA, House HP. Revision stapedectomy: A review of 258 cases. *Laryngoscope.* 1981;91:43–51.

Smyth GD, Kerr AG, Singh KP. Second ear stapedectomy: A continued controversy. *J Laryngol Otol.* 1975;89:1047–1056.

Vernick DM, Kartush JM. Revision stapedectomy with KTP and carbon dioxide (CO2) lasers. *Oper Tech Otolaryngol—Head Neck Surg.* 1998;9(2):82–87.

# Chapter 16

# Special Conditions and Complications in Otosclerosis Surgery

In this section we discuss common problems that could be encountered during stapedectomy surgery. Understanding these problems is helpful in providing a solution when dealing with these difficulties, especially when they are encountered during surgery. The occasional stapes surgeon as well as the experienced stapes surgeon could encounter these situations. The experienced stapes surgeon will be taxed when trying to restore hearing in the presence of various obstacles that are present.

## CEREBROSPINAL FLUID GUSHER

This complication is also known as a perilymph gusher, although in fact it is cerebrospinal fluid (CSF) that escapes. A CSF gusher occurs when the vestibule is opened and CSF gushes out. It is thought to be due to an abnormal patency of the cochlear aqueduct (Shea 1963) or to a defect in the fundus of the internal auditory canal (Schuknecht and Reisser 1988). A CSF gusher occurs rarely; it was reported in only 0.03% of cases by Causse and Causse (1980). Most cases of CSF gushers are associated with congenital fixation of the footplate in the pediatric population rather than in adults. Suzuki (1960) and Wlodyka (1978), however, showed that as age increases, so does the incidence of patency of the cochlear aqueduct. Farrior and Endicott (1971) reported two convincing cases where ablation of the cochlea aqueduct was required to control a CSF gusher, although author Glasscock (1973) reported the need to pack the vestibule in a CSF gusher because of a defect in the fundus of the internal auditory canal. Schuknecht and Reisser (1988) postulated that a widely patent cochlear aqueduct may be the etiology of an "oozer," whereas "gushers" are the result of defects in the fundus of the internal auditory canal.

### Can the Surgeon Be Alerted Prior to Surgery about the Presence of a Possible CSF Gusher?

A CT scan of the temporal bones can demonstrate the presence of an abnormally patent cochlear aqueduct or detect if a defect of the fundus exists. Two other clues can help alert the surgeon to the presence of a gusher

(Causse et al 1983): an avascular congenital middle ear and an abnormal anterior insertion of the posterior crus to the footplate.

## Management of a CSF Gusher

Management of a CSF gusher involves the following steps:

1. Elevation of the head

2. Lumbar spinal drain to remove as much CSF as possible

3. Small fenestra stapedotomy

4. Tissue seal over the fenestra is mandatory. Some experts recommend that a prosthesis be placed to keep the seal over the fenestra in place (Wiet et al 1993).

Complete control of the CSF gusher is necessary because this complication has the potential to cause meningitis. The patient's hearing is likely to deteriorate following such a complication. Some surgeons recommend drilling a small control hole in the footplate prior to creating an actual fenestra for stapedotomy. This is done to avoid a "cork in a bottle" effect when the vestibule is suddenly opened.

## MALLEUS FIXATION

Malleus fixation may result from ossification of the superior and anterior suspensory ligaments. The malleus head may be fixed congenitally. Approximately three fourths of malleus fixations are associated with stapedial otosclerosis. The incidence of malleus fixation is approximately 1%, as reported by most centers (Lippy and Schuring 1978; Powers et al 1967). Causse and Causse (1980), however, reported that malleus fixation occurs in as many as 10.6% of patients undergoing primary stapedectomy.

## Can Malleus Fixation Be Diagnosed Prior to Surgery?

Moon and Hahn (1981) offered several clues to diagnose the presence of malleus fixation:

1. Lack of movement of the manubrium and umbo on pneumatic otoscopy

2. Palpation of the malleus (on occasion, this may prove to be painful, however)

3. Audiologic findings that seldom reveal an air-bone gap of more than 30 dB

4. Acoustic reflexes with isolation of the tensor tympani on impedance audiometry. A jet of air is blown across the cornea or the tragus is stroked; if no readings are detected or if they are faint, it is likely that malleus fixation is present.

Vincent et al (1999) presented the following features by which malleus ankylosis may be suspected:

1. Unilateral mixed hearing loss that is usually nonprogressive

2. Small air-bone gap predominantly in the low frequencies

3. Association with sensorineural impairment in the high frequencies

4. Acoustic reflex absent on the impaired side but present in the contra-lateral ear

Moon and Hahn (1981) described an atrophic tympanic membrane that becomes flaccid while continuing to function against a fixed malleus handle. Many of these tympanic membranes return to normal once the ankylosis is repaired. Primary malleus fixation occurs late in life, whereas otosclerosis occurs mainly in young or middle-aged adults. A conductive hearing loss of 10 to 15 dB is more commonly seen with isolated malleus fixation (Powers et al 1967). Carhart's notch, which is typical of stapedial otosclerosis, can also be seen in malleus fixation as a result of ossicular inertia.

## Management

If the ossified ligaments are fractured, it is likely that they will get refixed. An incus bypass procedure using either an incus replacement prosthesis (IRP) or a total ossicular replacement prosthesis (TORP) has been advocated. The treatment lies in amputating the head of the malleus after removing the incus. The tympanic membrane is dissected off the handle of the malleus; an IRP is crimped over the handle and placed into the fenestra of the footplate. Sheehy (1982) recommended a TORP in these situations; Fisch et al (2001), however, recommended malleostapedotomy and have reported good results with this technique.

## Results

Sheehy (1982) reported that 64% of patients had closure to within 10 dB. Ninety-five percent of cases had a 20 dB or less residual conductive deficit. Results were the same whether an IRP or a TORP was used.

## INCUS PROBLEMS ENCOUNTERED DURING PRIMARY STAPES SURGERY

Problems include fusion of the incus to the malleus, accidental dislocation of the incus during surgery, congenital anomalies, and incudal necrosis.

Incus malleus fixation has a 1% reported incidence in association with otosclerosis (Moon and Hahn 1981). Fused malleus and incus are seen in congenital abnormalities of the ear. Postinflammatory changes such as tympanosclerosis, fibrosis, and adhesions can lead to fixation of the incus. An abnormally short or malformed incus may make it difficult to attach the prosthesis to it. One study presenting such features reported that an incus bypass procedure was required (Sheehy 1982). Overall incus problems (fixation, dislocation, and congenital abnormalities) are common indications for a bypass technique. When a bypass technique is undertaken, an IRP or a TORP is most commonly used; it is therefore necessary for the otolaryngologist to be able to perform such bypass techniques. Sheehy (1982) found that such bypass techniques were needed in 2% of primary stapedectomies.

## Management

If the incus is accidentally dislocated, it can be replaced without further problems, and the stapedectomy can proceed as usual (Causse and Causse 1980). Alternatively, the incus can be removed and an incus bypass procedure undertaken. An IRP or a TORP can be used in this situation.

## Necrosis of the Long Process of the Incus

Lippy and Schuring (1974) recommended a modified Robinson prosthesis, reporting excellent results with the use of this prosthesis.

## POSTOPERATIVE REPARATIVE GRANULOMA

Postoperative reparative granuloma is known to cause sensorineural hearing loss following stapedectomy.

## Incidence

Kaufman and Schuknecht (1967) found an incidence of 1.3% of cases that developed granuloma formation, and Harris and Weiss (1962) found an incidence of 5% in their series.

## Clinical Presentation

Sudden deterioration in hearing 1 to 6 weeks following surgery is suggestive of reparative granuloma. On inspection, the tympanic membrane appears reddish in color, especially at the posterior superior quadrant. Bone conduction and speech discrimination scores are affected. Kaufman and Shuknecht (1967) reported that in the majority of cases symptoms occurred in the first 3 weeks following surgery, and Gacek (1970) reported similar findings. Hearing loss is a typical finding. Vertigo was found to occur in 20 to 35% of cases. In some patients, tinnitus was present.

Some granulomas may occupy the middle ear without invading the vestibule, and these usually heal without catastrophic sequelae. Even though they may extend into the vestibule, they generally are not adherent to the saccule or utricle and can be safely removed (Pratt and Winchester 1962). Those that invade the vestibule, however, are accompanied by sensorineural hearing loss. Serous labyrinthitis is usually an accompanying feature. Such invasive granulomas are usually associated with fat or gelatin sponge being used as a seal on the fenestra created by the surgeon. Reparative granulomas are often found to engulf the prosthesis and long process of the incus, often in direct contact with the tympanic membrane.

## Audiological Findings

A pure tone threshold loss for bone conduction is a typical finding. A simultaneous conductive hearing loss may also be present; partly due to the mass effect of the granuloma and partly due to the fluid in the middle ear. There is a marked decrease of speech discrimination scores, usually with a score of 60% or less.

## Appearance of the Tympanic Membrane

The tympanic membrane is thickened, especially in the posterior half. On occasion, the tympanic membrane may even be edematous.

## Etiology

Granuloma is the result of nonsuppurative labyrinthitis in the open oval window. Granuloma formation is associated with total removal of the footplate and the use of gelatin sponge. It is rarely associated with small fenestra stapedotomy. Gacek (1970) associated gelatin sponge as an oval window seal with the formation of granuloma; Kaufman and Schuknecht (1967) also confirmed this. They found no evidence of infection. Tange and colleagues (Tange et al 2002) reviewed 475 stapes surgeries where a pure gold prosthesis was used. They found that in their series the incidence of reparative granuloma was 1.5%. Microscopic examination of granuloma demonstrates fibroblastic proliferation, numerous capillaries, chronic cell infiltrate, and foreign body giant cells.

Harris and Weiss (1962) demonstrated bone spicules, foreign body material such as cotton fibers, and keratin, and postulated that these might have been the cause of granulomas. Granuloma formation has also been associated with fat wire prosthesis, gelatin sponge (Gelfoam), and large fenestra stapedectomy (Beales 1981).

## Management

Early surgery, with removal of the granuloma and regrafting of the oval window and a change of the prosthesis, produces excellent results. Immediate recognition, along with immediate removal of the granuloma, offers the best chance to cure the ear of this problem, especially if it is removed before serous labyrinthitis has occurred. If it is treated promptly, hearing returns to normal. Gacek (1970) demonstrated that revision surgery with removal of the granuloma, when done in the first 2 weeks of presentation, results in good preservation of hearing even though speech discrimination scores may have fallen below 50%. The removal should be done at the earliest date because a delay of 2 weeks or more means the chances of a permanent residual deficit are high.

Immediate recognition of granuloma formation and timely surgery for removal of the granuloma also provide good results for the return of bone conduction thresholds, as well as relief from vertigo and tinnitus. If removal of the granuloma occurs prior to the onset of serofibrinous labyrinthitis, the prognosis is usually good.

## PERSISTENT STAPEDIAL ARTERY

The stapedial artery is a primitive vessel structure that normally atrophies during the third month of human fetal life. Hyrtl first reported persistence of the stapedial artery in 1836. The stapedial artery arises from the internal carotid artery, enters the middle ear in the anteroinferior quadrant, passes over the promontory, proceeds through the obturator foramen of the stapes, and turns anteriorly into the horizontal portion of the facial canal through a bony dehiscence. Subsequently it enters the middle cranial fossa and terminates in the middle meningeal artery. The stapedial artery has two major divisions: the dorsal (supraorbital) and the ventral (maxillomandibular). The supraorbital division undergoes anastomosis with the ophthalmic artery and is incorporated into the anterior branch of the middle meningeal artery. The maxillomandibular division undergoes anastomosis with the internal maxillary branch of the external carotid artery, supplying the lower face, inferior alveolar, and infraorbital regions.

Usually the stem of the stapedial artery atrophies, and the anastomosis with the external carotid artery takes over the blood supply of both divisions. If the transition fails to take place, the middle meningeal artery will be supplied by the ophthalmic artery or a persistent stapedial artery.

## Incidence

The reported incidence of persistent stapedial artery is about 1 in 5000 to 10,000 ears (House and Patterson 1964; Marion et al 1985). Moreano and colleagues (1994) reported 5 cases of temporal bone study in 1025 ears (0.48%). The reported incidence of persistent stapedial artery during surgery was lower, in the range of 0.02% (Steffen 1968) to 0.05% (David 1967).

## Can a Persistent Stapedial Artery Be Diagnosed before Surgery?

Theoretically, a persistent stapedial artery can cause pulsatile tinnitus. It may also present with a conductive hearing loss by limiting stapes movement. Sensorineural hearing loss, probably caused by erosion of the bony otic capsule, has been reported (Kelemen 1958). A persistent stapedial artery can be associated with internal carotid artery or middle ear anomalies, especially with anomalies of the stapes and facial nerve (Tien and Linthicum 2001). It has been associated infrequently with trisomy 13, 15 syndrome, second branchial arch anomaly, Paget's disease, otosclerosis, and thalidomide deformities (Boscia et al 1990).

## Treatment

The most important clinical significance of persistent stapedial artery is the possibility of bleeding from injury to the vessel during the course of stapedectomy. Treatment of a persistent stapedial artery identified during the course of stapedectomy, however, is not well established. There is a theoretical risk of hemiplegia if the vessel is clamped. In fact, the embryonic origin has caused surgeons in the past to fear complications such as contralateral hemiplegia. This fear has caused some surgeons to abandon stapedectomy altogether (Diamond 1987; Govaerts et al 1993). If a persistent stapedial artery is identified, then as atraumatic surgery as possible should be performed, with due care being accorded to the vessel.

In 12 reported cases of persistent stapedial artery with associated footplate ankylosis, 11 patients underwent stapedectomy (Horn and Visvanathan 1998). In nine cases in which a prosthesis was placed, there were no postoperative complications. In five of these nine cases, the artery was sectioned or clipped without complication. Horn and Visvanathan thus concluded that successful stapedectomy can be performed even in the presence of a persistent stapedial artery.

The persistent stapedial artery causes horizontal obscuring of the oval window. The first important step is removal of the stapes superstructure without damaging the artery. The laser is a suitable tool for this step. Fenestration of the footplate should also be accomplished with minimal trauma. Again, the laser is a suitable tool for this. Horn and Visvanathan (1998) noted that the artery lies closer to the anterior crus than to the posterior crus; they recommended the Causse prosthesis in this situation because it is smooth and less likely to traumatize the artery.

## FLOATING FOOTPLATE

Floating footplate can occur when the footplate is not properly fixed and becomes mobilized. It is most likely to occur if a fenestra is placed in the center. Some experts recommend creating a control hole in the footplate before removing the arch of the stapes. If it is not possible to remove the footplate atraumatically or efficiently, surgery should be abandoned, and a soft tissue seal should be placed over the oval window. Some reports in the literature advocate applying a vein graft above the floating footplate, then attaching a prosthesis from the incus to the floating footplate if it remains hinged inward (Lippy and Schuring 1973, 1983). Good results have been reported with this technique. If the mobilized footplate is mostly blue with diffuse otosclerosis, then the success rate is 95% (Lippy 1994). If the footplate is thick, white, or biscuit shaped, the hearing success rate is approximately 52%. Should the footplate mobilize again during revision surgery, no further surgery should be planned. Lippy (1994) stated that when he followed this protocol, none of the 147 patients who developed a floating footplate in a series of 8000 cases developed a sensorineural hearing loss.

Should it not be possible to proceed with surgery, and if further attempts are made to remove the footplate, this could result in further submerging the footplate, with resulting sensorineural hearing loss. Surgery in such cases should be abandoned.

A floating footplate is less likely to be encountered when a laser is used to create a fenestra. Should a floating footplate be encountered and no laser is available, then Perkins (1994) recommended that the procedure be halted and reoperation be considered only after a period of 4 months. This should be adequate time to allow the footplate to get refixed. The laser is best used for such a condition, and a vein clad prosthesis is used.

Other surgical procedures advocated for a floating footplate are to create a pothole in the promontory near the footplate, then lift and remove the submerged footplate (House 1963). In a poll conducted by Wiet et al (1993) on a strategy regarding a floating footplate, the plurality of respondents (45%) advocated removal of the footplate, and a minority (12%) stated that they would terminate the procedure. One third said that they would place a prosthesis with or without a seal on the oval window. When polled about a submerged footplate, 71% stated that they would leave the footplate alone, and 29% stated that they would attempt removal.

## DEHISCENT (PTOTIC) FACIAL NERVE

Fowler (1961), Basek (1962), and Proctor and Nager (1982) summarized the course of the facial nerve and its variations within the temporal bone. A common anomaly is failure of osseous closure of the fallopian canal by the otic capsule. Baxter (1971) reported an incidence of 55% of bony dehiscence of the fallopian canal. A minor dehiscence of the fallopian canal does not lead to a ptotic facial nerve.

Durcan et al (1967) hypothesized that inferior displacement of the facial nerve is most likely due to an arrest or anomaly of Reichert's cartilage. Durcan et al also described three anomalies of the facial nerve in relationship to the oval window: an overhanging facial nerve, a bifid facial nerve, and a facial nerve coursing over the promontory. They postulated that failure of Reichert's cartilage to make contact with the lateral wall of the cartilaginous otic capsule leads to a ptotic facial nerve; this results in an anomalous stapes arch that does not contact the otic capsule. The absence of the normal stapes superstructure allows the facial nerve to develop at or below the level of the oval window. The bifid facial nerve is caused by the late union of Reichert's cartilage to the otic capsule. Usually, under these circumstances, the stapes crura are atrophic, and the anterior crura is frequently absent.

Welling et al (1992) found that when facial nerve anomalies are present, they do not occur alone but are part of a continuum of anomalies. Horn and Visvanathan (1998) offered the options of abandoning the procedure, fenestration, facial nerve decompression with displacement from the oval window, or cochleotomy, for dealing with the ptotic facial nerve when treating otosclerosis. De La Cruz and Chandrasekhar (1994) wrote that fenestration under these circumstances is appropriate because usually there is a lateral ossicular chain anomaly that accompanies this disorder. In cases where there is partial ptosis of the facial nerve, the nerve may be gently retracted, and the surgeon can proceed with stapedectomy. If there are several anomalies present, however, it is advisable that the surgeon terminate the procedure immediately.

## DYSGEUSIA AND AGEUSIA

Most surgeons try to preserve the chorda tympani. Once the annnulus of the tympanic membrane is elevated and the middle ear is entered, the next step should be to locate the chorda tympani. The chorda tympani is then elevated out up to the handle of the malleus. Care should be taken not to stretch the nerve. If the chorda is allowed to dry out, taste disturbances last approximately 4 to 5 months but generally disappear without treatment. Should the chorda tympani obstruct vision (in very rare instances), it is better to section the nerve rather than stretch it. Should taste disturbances persist and prove a problem to the patient for 6 months or more following stapedectomy, then the nerve should be sectioned.

## FACIAL PARALYSIS

Unfortunately, facial paralysis can occur. If the facial nerve is dehiscent, and the surgeon is experienced and confident that he or she has not damaged the nerve, the nerve can be expected to recover. If the nerve has been damaged, then decompression may be required. On occasion, the facial palsy may be a result of the local anesthetic, in which case, the facial nerve recovers within 24 hours.

## CHOLESTEATOMA FORMATION POSTSTAPEDECTOMY

Fortunately, cholesteatoma formation is a rare occurrence. The surgeon needs to take proper care to prevent implantation of stratified keratinizing squamous epithelium in the middle ear. If the cholesteatoma is small, it can be removed without affecting the stapedectomy; if the cholesteatoma is large, however, then it needs to be attended to. The surgeon may need to remove the prosthesis after weighing the risks with the patient.

Mechanisms by which cholesteatoma can occur following stapedectomy are chronic eustachian tube dysfunction and negative middle ear pressures. Fergusson et al (1986) reported on how cholesteatoma can occur: if the prosthesis extrudes, it provides a portal through which keratinizing stratified squamous epithelium can enter the middle ear. On occasion, an attic retraction pocket can grow into a cholesteatoma. Cholesteatoma can also occur if stratified squamous epithelium has been inadvertently implanted into the middle ear. Cholesteatoma can also occur from an improperly positioned tympanomeatal flap, as well as from a marginal perforation where the annulus has been disrupted. Once cholesteatoma formation has occurred, it must be dealt with appropriately because it has the potential not only to destroy hearing but also to cause life-threatening meningitis.

## TYMPANIC MEMBRANE PERFORATION

The tympanic membrane may be perforated during surgery. This can be repaired immediately and simultaneously with perichondrium or with a vein graft. This is done by underlay technique and is nearly always successful.

Perforation of the tympanic membrane nearly always occurs when elevating the tympanomeatal flap. Careful identification of the annulus will help avoid this complication. Damage to the tympanic membrane has been reported in 1.9% of cases by Causse and Causse (1980).

## REFERENCES

Basek M. Anomalies of the facial nerve in normal temporal bones. *Ann Otol, Rhinol Laryngol.* 1962;71:382–390.

Baxter A. Dehiscence of the fallopian canal. *J Laryngol Otol.* 1971;85:587–594.

Beales PH. Hearing loss after stapedectomy. In: *Otosclerosis.* Bristol: John Wright and Sons; 1981:169–185.

Boscia R, Knox RD, Adkins WY, Holgate RC. Persistent stapedial artery supplying a glomus tympanicum tumor. *Arch Otolaryngol—Head Neck Surg.* 1990;116:852–854.

Causse JB, Causse JR, Wiet RJ, Yoo TJ. Complications of stapedectomies. *Am J Otolaryngol.* 1983;4:275–280.

Causse JR, Causse JB. Eighteen year report on stapedectomy I: Problems of stapedial fixation. *Clin Otolaryngol.* 1980;5:49–59.

David GD. Persistent stapedial artery: A temporal bone report. *J Laryngol Otol.* 1967;81:649–660.

De La Cruz A, Chandrasekhar SS. Congenital malformation of the temporal bone. In: Brackmann DE, Shelton C, Arriaga MA, eds. *Otologic Surgery.* Philadelphia: WB Saunders; 1994:69–84.

Diamond MK. Unusual example of a persistent stapedial artery in a human. *Anat Record.* 1987;218:345–354.

Durcan DJ, Shea JJ, Sleeckx JP. Bifurcation of the facial nerve. *Arch Otolaryngol.* 1967; 86:37–49.

Farrior B, Endicott JN. Congenital mixed deafness: Cerebrospinal fluid otorrhea: Ablation of the aqueduct of the cochlea. *Laryngoscope.* 1971;81:684–699.

Fergusson BJ, Gillespie CA, Kenan PD, Farmer JC. Mechanisms of cholesteatoma formation following stapedectomy. *Am J Otolaryngol.* 1986;7(6):420–424.

Fisch U, Acar GO, Huber AM. Malleostapedotomy ion revision surgery for otosclerosis. *Otol Neurotol.* 2001;22:776–785.

Fowler EP. Variations in the temporal bone course of the facial nerve. *Laryngoscope.* 1961;71:937–946.

Gacek RR. The diagnosis and treatment of poststapedectomy granuloma. *Am J Otolaryngol.* 1970;7:420–424.

Glasscock ME. The stapes gusher. *Arch Otolaryngol.* 1973;98:82–91.

Govaerts PJ, Cremers WRJ, Marquet TF, et al. Persistent stapedial artery: Does it prevent successful surgery? *Ann Otol, Rhinol Laryngol.* 1993;102:724–728.

Harris I, Weiss L. Granulomatous complications of oval window fat grafts. *Laryngoscope.* 1962;72:870–885.

Horn KL, Visvanathan A. Stapes surgery in the obscured oval window: Management of the ptotic facial nerve and the persistent stapedial artery. *Oper Tech Otolaryngol—Head Neck Surg.* 1998;9(1):58–63.

House HP. Early and late complications of stapes surgery. *Arch Otolaryngol.* 1963; 78:606–613.

House HP, Patterson ME. Persistent stapedial artery: A report of two cases. *Trans Am Acad Ophthalmol Otolaryngol.* 1964;68:644–646.

Kaufman RS, Schuknecht HF. Reparative granuloma following stapedectomy: A clinical entity. *Ann Otol, Rhinol Laryngol.* 1967;76:1008–1017.

Kelemen GD. Arteria stapedial in bilateral persistence. *Arch Otolaryngol.* 1958;67: 668–677.

Lippy WH. Special problems of otosclerosis surgery. In: Brackmann DE, Shelton CS, Arriaga M, eds. *Otologic Surgery.* Philadelphia: WB Saunders; 1994:348–355.

Lippy WH, Schuring A. Treatment of the inadvertently mobilized footplate. *Arch Otolaryngol—Head Neck Surg.* 1973;98:80–81.

Lippy WH, Schuring AG. Prostheses for the problem incus in stapedectomy. *Arch Otolaryngol.* 1974;100:237–239.

Lippy WH, Schuring AG. Stapedectomy for otosclerosis with malleus fixation. *Arch Otolaryngol.* 1978;98:80–81.

Lippy WH, Schuring A. Solving ossicular problems in stapedectomy. *Laryngoscope.* 1983;93:1147–1150.

Marion J, Hinojosa R, Khan AA. Persistent stapedial artery: A histopathologic study. *Otolaryngol Head Neck Surg.* 1985;93:298–312.

Moon CN, Hahn MJ. Primary malleus fixation: Diagnosis and treatment. *Laryngoscope.* 1981;91:1298–1306.

Moreano EH, Paparella MM, Zelterman D, Goycoolea MV. Prevalence of facial canal dehiscence and of persistent stapedial artery in the human middle ear: A report of 1,000 temporal bones. *Laryngoscope.* 1994;104:309–320.

Perkins R. Laser stapedotomy. In: Brackmann DE, Shelton CS, Arriaga M, eds. *Otologic Surgery.* Philadelphia: WB Saunders; 1994:314–329.

Powers WH, Sheehy JL, House HP. The fixed malleus head: A report of 35 cases. *Arch Otolaryngol.* 1967;85:177–181.

Pratt LL, Winchester RA. Fibromatous polyp of the vestibule. *Arch Otolaryngol.* 1962; 75:98–102.

Proctor B, Nager GT. The facial canal: Normal anatomy, variations and anomalies. *Ann Otol, Rhinol Laryngol.* 1982;91(suppl 93):33–61.

Schuknecht HF, Reisser C. The morphologic basis for perilymph gushers and oozers. *Arch Otorhinolaryngol.* 1988;39:1–12.

Shea JJ. Complications of the stapedectomy operation. *Ann Otol, Rhinol Laryngol.* 1963;72:1109–1123.

Sheehy JL. Stapedectomy: Incus bypass procedures—a report of 203 operations. *Laryngoscope.* 1982;92:258–262.

Steffen TN. Vascular anomalies of the middle ear. *Laryngoscope.* 1968;78:171–197.

Suzuki T. A study on the communication between labyrinth and cerebrospinal space through cochlear aqueduct in human body. *J Otolaryngol (Japan).* 1960;63: 2298–2312.

Tange RA, Schimanski G, Van Lange JW, Grolman W, Zuur LC. Reparative granuloma seen in cases of gold piston implantation after stapes surgery for otosclerosis. *Auris, Nasus, Larynx.* 2002;29(1):7–10.

Tien HC, Linthicum FH. Persistent stapedial artery. *Otol Neurotol* 2001;22(6):975–976.

Vincent R, Lopez A, Sperling NM. Malleus ankylosis: A clinical, audiometric, histologic and surgical study of 123 cases. *Am J Otolaryngol.* 1999;20:717–725.

Welling DB, Glasscock ME, Gantz BJ. Avulsion of the facial nerve at stapedectomy. *Laryngoscope.* 1992;102:729–733.

Wiet RJ, Harvey SA, Bauer GP. Complications in stapes surgery: Options for prevention and management. *Otolaryngol Clin N Am.* 1993;26:471–490.

Wlodyka J. Studies on cochlear aqueduct patency. *Ann Otol, Rhinol Laryngol.* 1978;87:22–28.

**167**

# Chapter *17*

# Otodystrophies

The otodystrophies are a group of disorders that affect the temporal bone and the otic capsule. Most of these disorders, unlike otosclerosis, affect not only the otic capsule but other areas of the temporal bone as well, in addition to involving other bones of the body. It is important to know that they can present as conductive deafness and that the audiometric configuration can resemble that of otosclerosis.

## OSTEOGENESIS IMPERFECTA

Osteogenesis imperfecta is a rare bone disorder. It represents a group of heterogeneous systemic connective tissue disorders that predispose the individual to recurrent fractures when subjected to trivial trauma.

### Incidence of Osteogenesis Imperfecta

The incidence of osteogenesis imperfecta varies between 2 and 15 per 100,000 births (Pedersen 1985). It is a hereditary disorder of collagen synthesis and occurs in two main forms, osteogenesis imperfecta congenital (OIC) and osteogenesis imperfecta tarda (OIT). In the congenital form, fractures occur in utero, and the fetus dies. In the tarda form, fractures often occur following minor trivial trauma during childhood. This becomes less frequent, however, with the onset of adolescence. Malalignment of the fractured bones leads to deformities and excessive callus formation. OIT has a dominant mode of inheritance, with variable penetrance with asymptomatic carriers, although cases without a family history of OIT are known to occur.

### Signs and Symptoms of Osteogenesis Imperfecta

The cardinal features of this disease are fractures that occur following relatively minor trivial, often unrecognized trauma. Approximately 50 to 60% of patients eventually develop a hearing loss, and 85% have blue sclera (Quisiling et al 1979). Blue sclerae are also associated with collagen disorders such as Ehlers-Danlos syndrome and Marfan's syndrome.

The symptom complex that includes multiple fractures, blue sclerae, and deafness is known as van der Hoeve's and de Kleyn's syndrome. The syndrome was described earlier by Adair Dighton (1912) and Bronson (1917). It was also noticed, however, that in some family members, hearing impairment and blue sclerae presented without the tendency for fractures.

Altered collagen synthesis results in defective connective tissue, with a tendency to hypermobility and laxity of joints, thin skin, and easy bruising in the subcutaneous tissues. The teeth of these patients are abnormal in approximately 15% of cases. The dentine is abnormal, or the enamel is cracked, resulting in yellow-stained, irregular teeth. This is known as amelogenesis imperfecta.

The clinical course of OIT is variable. Sillence et al (1979) introduced a classification based on genetic and clinical criteria. Type 1 is autosomal dominant, mild, and manifested by blue sclerae. Type 2 is autosomal dominant or recessive and is uniformly lethal. Type 3 is autosomal recessive and is marked by progressive skeletal deformities, with extreme fragility of bones and very short stature. Type 4 is autosomal dominant and is intermediate with patients exhibiting skeletal fragility and short stature.

## Otological Features of Osteogenesis Imperfecta

Hearing loss has long been recognized as a common feature in osteogenesis imperfecta and other otodystrophies (Table 17–1). The data in some publications could be taken to imply that with advancing age, the number of patients suffering from osteogenesis imperfecta approaches 100%. The typical feature of osteogenesis imperfecta is hearing loss that occurs in childhood, then rapidly progresses. The incidence of deafness in childhood is between 10 and 20%; by middle age, approximately 50% of patients suffering from osteogenesis imperfecta will also be suffering from deafness. The hearing loss may increase during pregnancy. The audiometric pattern of hearing loss is indistinguishable from that of otosclerosis. Typically, the hearing loss commences at puberty, when fractures become less frequent.

A conductive hearing loss is present in nearly 80% of cases. Very often a mixed hearing loss is present. On occasion, a purely sensorineural hearing loss may be present, and on rare occasions profound irreversible sensorineural hearing loss is present (Pedersen 1985; Shapiro et al 1982; Stewart and O'Reilly 1989). Sensorineural hearing loss in OIT is believed to be due to encroachment of reparative vascular and fibrous tissue in and about the cochlea or as the result of microfractures and/or hemorrhages (Shapiro et al 1982). Several studies have indicated that the incidence of hearing loss of both types increases with age, as does the proportion of patients with mixed types (Garretsen et al 1997). In one study (Stewart and O'Reilly 1989), 11 out of 12 patients between ages 40 and 49 were affected, as were all 7 patients between 50 and 55 years of age.

Table 17–1  Clinical Manifestations of the Otodystrophies

|  | CHL | SNHL | FND |
|---|---|---|---|
| Fibrous dysplasia | common | uncommon | uncommon |
| Paget's disease | common | very common | uncommon |
| Osteogenesis imperfecta | common | uncommon | rare |
| Osteopetrosis | common | common | common. |

CHL = conductive hearing loss; FND = facial nerve dysfunction; SNHL = sensorineural hearing loss.

In a study involving 1394 patients with osteogenesis imperfecta (Paterson et al 2001), the most common age of onset was from the second to the fourth decade of life. The investigators found that at age 50, approximately half of the patients in their series had symptoms of hearing impairment.

Tympanometry shows increased compliance values. Stapes fixation is almost always associated with a conductive hearing loss. Hypermobility of the tympanic membrane can be seen simultaneously with fractures or aplasia of the crura of the stapes. Hypermobility of the tympanic membrane occurs because the tympanic membrane has the same embryological origin as the sclera. In those patients who have fractures of the stapedial arch, high compliance values are seen on tympanometry. Carhart's notches are not present, nor is Schwartze's sign. Usually the conductive hearing losses are not bilateral, but if and when bilateral conductive hearing losses are present, they are not symmetrical.

Vestibular symptoms are rare in osteogenesis imperfecta (Shea and Postma 1982). Johnsson and colleagues (1982), however, have described extensive bilateral endolymphatic hydrops in a patient who suffered from osteogenesis imperfecta.

## Histology of Osteogenesis Imperfecta

Deposition of osteopenic immature bony tissue that is weak is characteristic of osteogenesis imperfecta. Often, microfractures can be found. Histologically, the number of osteocytes is increased in both woven and lamellar bone accompanied by a relative reduction of matrix substance. The bone turnover rate is very high. OIT has multiorgan manifestations such as fragile bones, hearing loss, dentinogenesis imperfecta, loose joints, mitral valve prolapse, easy bruising, and growth deficiency (Bergstrom 1977; Marini 1988).

Although there are some similarities between otosclerosis and osteogenesis imperfecta, both are separate and distinct entities, with defects in the stapes as seen in osteogenesis imperfecta being quite different from those seen in otosclerosis (Berger et al 1986; Pedersen et al 1985). Biochemical analysis of stapes sulfhydryl groups and various enzymes have clearly demonstrated different concentrations in both of these diseases (Arslan and Ricci 1963; Chevance 1964; Holdsworth et al 1973). In most cases, stapedial fixation is caused by a focal lesion in the footplate that histologically resembles the early active stage of otosclerosis. On occasion, fixation of the stapedial footplate is the result of diffuse structural alteration of the entire footplate. The extensive degree of disorganization is more pronounced in osteogenesis imperfecta than in otosclerosis (Brosnan et al 1977). Biochemical assays of serum calcium, phosphorus, and calciferol are normal. Alkaline phosphatase levels occasionally may be elevated. Photon absorptiometry has demonstrated that the cortical thickness of bone is reduced; this is not seen in otosclerosis.

## Radiological Findings of Osteogenesis Imperfecta

Temporal bone findings in OIT are nearly identical to those in otosclerosis (Table 17–2). Diffuse resorption of vast areas of the otic capsule is commonly seen in OIT. In advanced cases of OIT, the middle ear cleft can become narrowed by proliferative bone, and the oval and round windows can be obliterated by the dysplastic process.

**Table 17–2  Radiological Findings in the Otodystrophies**

|  | EAC stenosis | IAC stenosis | ME | OC |
|---|---|---|---|---|
| Fibrous dysplasia | present | rare | rare | uninvolved |
| Paget's disease | absent | absent | rare | uninvolved |
| Osteogenesis imperfecta | absent | absent | rare | rare |
| Osteopetrosis | present | present | present | involved |

EAC = external auditory canal; IAC = internal auditory canal; ME = middle ear involvement; OC = otic capsule.

## Treatment of Osteogenesis Imperfecta

At this time, there is no known cure for OIT. Treatment is instead directed at rehabilitation, although medical treatment for OIT remains elusive. Calcitonin, sodium fluoride, and vitamin D have each been found to have poor efficacy.

## Role of Stapedectomy in Osteogenesis Imperfecta

Results of stapedectomy are generally satisfactory (Armstrong 1984) and are similar to those of otosclerosis (Garretsen and Cremers 1990). Stapedectomy, however, should be delayed until well into adulthood (Pederson and Elbrond 1983). By then it is expected that fractures in response to trivial trauma will have ceased (Kosoy and Maddox 1971).

The findings of the middle ear include a very thick and soft footplate. The middle ear mucosa appears to be more vascular than normal. There is a high chance of floating footplate. The long process of the incus may be fragile and prone to fracture during crimping. Other findings include thin canal wall skin, brittle scutum, and fragile stapedial crura.

## PAGET'S DISEASE (OSTEITIS DEFORMANS)

Paget's disease is characterized by excessive remodeling of bone. This disorder typically affects the axial skeleton. Pathognomonic features of Paget's are spreading osteolytic and osteoblastic changes that commonly affect the pelvis, lumbar spine, skull, femur, and tibia. The typical patient suffering from Paget's disease has an enlarged skull, progressive kyphosis, bowed legs, and short stature.

## Incidence of Paget's Disease

Males are four times more likely to be affected than females. The geographic distribution of Paget's disease includes a large concentration of patients in the United Kingdom, Australia, and New Zealand (Detheridge et al 1982). Paget's disease can occur sporadically, but in 15% of cases there is an autosomal dominant inheritance pattern (Avioli 1987). Very rarely does the onset of this disease occur before the age of 40; it is commonly encountered after the age of 55. The overall incidence is 3% but increases by the eighth decade (Freeman 1988).

Only 20% of patients suffering from Paget's disease are symptomatic. The diagnosis is often made when the patient undergoes a routine health checkup. Recent reports implicate an immunoregulatory defect on chromosome 6. This finding, along with the identification of nuclear viral inclusions in osteoclasts, is suggestive of a viral etiology as a causative factor of Paget's dsease (Mills and Singer 1976). In Paget's disease, there is a chance of malignancy in about 2% of patients (Swartz and Harnsberger 1992).

## Histology of Paget's Disease

Alternating waves of osteoclastic and osteoblastic activity result in haphazard bony resorption followed by deposition of structurally weakened demineralized bone. In the early phase of the disease, bone resorption is accelerated and can be seen radiologically as a lytic area. The marrow then gets filled with fibrovascular tissue that later becomes sclerotic. The sclerosis contains a mosaic pattern of coarse fibers that are composed of irregularly arranged units of bone (Nager 1975).

## Nonotologic Features of Paget's Disease

The pelvis is the site that is most commonly involved, followed by the skull. The superficial temporal artery becomes hypertrophied and tortuous. Bone pain is a common symptom. Expansion of bone in and around the foramina can lead to neurologic deficits that can result in manifestations such as hemifacial spasm, trigeminal neuralgia, and optic atrophy (Clarke and Harrison 1978). Spinal cord lesions with vertebral involvement, nerve compression, and vascular steal syndrome are seen with Paget's disease. Ataxia, quadriparesis, hydrocephalus, and lower cranial nerve deficits can also occur (Davies 1968).

## Otologic Features of Paget's Disease

In many instances, a hearing loss is the only sign of Paget's disease; thus, the diagnosis can be missed. It is very uncommon for the temporal bone to be the only bone involved in Paget's (Lando et al 1988); however, involvement of both temporal bones along with other bones of the skull is common (Nager 1975). Of these patients, tinnitus and vertigo are seen in 20% of cases (Gutman and Kasabach 1936). The skull is involved in 65 to 70% of cases (Collins 1956). Hearing losses are seen in 30 to 50% of patients with involvement of the skull by Paget's disease of the bone (Nager 1975). The type of hearing loss was usually found to be a mixed hearing loss (Lindsay and Perlman 1936).

The etiology of hearing loss in Paget's disease remains unclear. Temporal bone findings as reported by Khetarpal and Schuknecht (1990) include stenosis of the eternal auditory canal, abnormalities of the tympanic membrane, tympanic cavity fibrosis, fixation of the stapes, and obliteration of the round window niche. These can explain the presence of a conductive hearing loss. Khetarpal and Schuknecht explained the sensorineural component of the hearing loss by reporting findings such as hair cell loss, arteriovenous shunts, otic capsule microfractures, stenosis of the internal auditory canal, and microneuromata. They postulated that the motion of mechanical elements in the middle and inner ears was in some way dampened by the bony dysplasia.

Other temporal bone findings as reported by Davies (1970), Nager (1975), and Proops et al (1985) include a tortuous external auditory canal, middle ear cleft constriction as a result of the remodeling response, remodeling of the ossicular chain with fixation of the ossicles, and otic capsule demineralization. Otic capsule invasion occurs from outer to inner fashion: the periosteal layer is first invaded, gradually progressing until the endosteal layer is involved. As the disease progresses, all the layers of the otic capsule are replaced (Lindsay and Suga 1976). When the endosteal layer becomes involved, usually the membranous labyrinth is obliterated (Lindsay and Lehman 1969). This pattern of otic capsule demineralization is in sharp contrast to the endochondral erosion of the bony labyrinth as seen in otosclerosis. An associated finding of the obliteration of the otic capsule is the demineralization of the petrous apex. Narrowing of the internal auditory canal is also accompanied by sensorineural hearing loss.

## Radiological Imaging of the Temporal Bone

The typical appearance of Paget's disease as seen on conventional x-rays is a "cotton wool" image caused by the coexistence of osteolysis and sclerosis. CT scanning of the temporal bone reflects the stage of activity of the temporal bone remodeling. The appearance can be divided into two broad categories: mosaic and translucent. The mosaic pattern demonstrates areas of radiolucency adjacent to foci of irregular sclerosis. A solitary cystic lucency may be the presenting feature in the early phase, and as the disease progresses, the mosaic pattern emerges.

In the translucent variant, the appearance of the temporal bone is homogeneous and diffusely blurred. Typically, the otic capsule's margins are blurred, and they are usually accompanied by diffuse demineralization of the petrous pyramid. The internal acoustic meatus, the external auditory canal, and the middle ear cleft are all likely to be stenotic and tortuous due to the disease process. Solitary involvement of the temporal bone by Paget's disease is rare. Paget's typically involves the axial skeleton, with typical radiographic features of sclerosis and lucencies that are flame shaped.

When the temporal bone is involved and demonstrates a mosaic pattern, it may be hard to distinguish it from fibrous dysplasia. This can sometimes pose a diagnostic dilemma. Under these circumstances, a biopsy may be needed to confirm the diagnosis. Solitary lucencies of the temporal bone can be caused by eosinophilic granuloma, infection, atypical fibrous dysplasia, metastatic disease, and malignant degeneration (Nager et al 1982).

## Management of Paget's Disease

Treatment of Paget's disease is with medication. Calcitonin has been shown to cause improvement clinically (Haddad et al 1970). Reversal of biochemical changes in response to calcitonin are also seen (Shai et al 1971). Other medications used are sodium etidronate (Smith et al 1971) and mithramycin (Elias and Evans 1972; Ryan et al 1980).

Serum alkaline phosphatase and urinary hydroxyproline are indicators of bone turnover activity and thus serve as useful indices to gauge the therapeutic response to treatment. Successful treatment results in a fall in the serum alkaline phosphatase and in urinary hydroxyproline excretion. Radiological imaging can also be used to gauge a patient's response to treatment.

Calcitonin causes a rapid inhibition of osteoblastic activity. When treatment is continued, it leads to a reduction in the rapid turnover of calcium and a gradual remineralization of bone. Calcitonin is usually given subcutaneously, but in recent times it has also been given intranasally via an aerosol (Gagel et al 1988; Reginster et al 1985). Calcitonin appears to be particularly effective when a neurologic complication has occurred in Paget's disease; especially when there is brainstem or spinal cord compression (De Rose et al 1974). Lando et al (1988) reported encouraging results when calcitonin was used as treatment for hearing loss in Paget's disease. A typical protocol consists of daily subcutaneous injections of 10 to 50 mg of calcitonin, which can be reduced to an alternate day regimen once serum alkaline phosphatase and urinary hydroxyproline return to normal.

Disodium etidronate (diphosphonate) is selectively concentrated in bone (Russell and Fleisch 1975). They inhibit calcium deposition and have selective toxicity for osteoclasts. Disodium etidronate can be given orally. Lando et al (1988) showed that a combination of calcitonin and disodium etidronate stabilizes hearing and in two cases reversed hearing loss associated with Paget's disease. A combination of calcitonin and disodium etidronate appears to be a promising modality of treatment for Paget's.

## Role of Stapedectomy in Paget's Disease

The results of stapedectomy have been reported to be poor in Paget's disease (Davies1968); thus, stapedectomy is not the surgical procedure of choice (Sparrow and Duval 1967). Modern hearing aids (Uppal et al 2001) have been reported to be better suited for this disease. It should be remembered that the disease process should first be stabilized before any hearing aids are given.

## OSTEOPETROSES

These are a group of inheritable metabolic disorders and are characterized by diffuse, dense sclerosis and abnormal bone remodeling. The osteopetrotic bone is immature, thick, dense, and brittle. This appearance gave rise to the terms *chalk* and *marble* bone disease. Two types have been identified:

1. The congenital or lethal form, which is autosomal recessive and makes itself evident during infancy. In the congenital form, there is medullary bony overgrowth, which causes obliteration of the marrow cavity. This in turn results in progressive pancytopenia. Death usually results, because the child is then unable to combat even simple infections. Few patients survive to adulthood (Hammersma 1970; Miyamoto et al 1980).

2. The tarda (adult) form is mostly autosomal dominant and on occasion is autosomal recessive. It is also known as Albers-Schönberg disease. The adult form has a variable clinical course, with up to 40% of patients being asymptomatic (Johnston et al 1968). The diagnosis is often made incidentally following an x-ray taken for other reasons.

The pathogenesis of osteopetrosis is incompletely understood, although the basic defect revolves around a defect of bone remodeling. A primary defect in osteoclast function has been hypothesized as the cause of osteopetrosis (Walker 1973, 1975a, 1975b).

## Clinical Features of the Osteopetroses

Clinical features of the osteopetroses are related to the progressive stenosis, with the resulting compression of the contents of the various foramina through which the cranial nerves exit the skull. In congenital osteopetrosis, Johnston et al (1968) found optic atrophy, facial nerve palsy, and hearing loss to be present in a significant number of patients. In the adult onset type of osteopetrosis, cranial nerve compression was also present in a large number of patients. Temporal bone findings usually demonstrate exuberant bony replacement by the dysplastic process, with crowding and narrowing of the middle ear cleft.

## Radiological Imaging of the Osteopetroses

Conventional x-rays demonstrate diffuse chalky sclerosis and thickening of the skull. Bollerslev and Andersen (1988) and Bollerslev et al (1988) suggested classifications based on the radiological appearances. Type 1 is manifested radiologically as diffuse sclerosis of the entire skull. Type 1 is associated with a high incidence of dysfunction of the fifth cranial nerve and a conductive hearing loss; type 1 is also associated with stenosis of the external and internal auditory canals. In type 2, the cranial base is extensively sclerotic and is accompanied by end plate thickening of the spine. Patients with type 2 osteopetrosis also exhibit facial nerve dysfunction.

CT scanning is an important tool for diagnosing this condition, and the typical dense chalky sclerotic lesions are pathognomonic of this condition.

## Management of the Osteopetroses

There is no effective medical treatment for this condition. Stapedectomy has no role. Hearing impairment is usually addressed by amplification. Surgery may be needed for recontouring of the external auditory canal if the external auditory canal is distorted by this disease. Should facial nerve dysfunction be present, total facial nerve decompression has been recommended (Dort et al 1990).

# FIBROUS DYSPLASIA

Fibrous dysplasia is a common, gradually progressive benign fibro-osseous disorder. The exact etiology is unknown, and it frequently halts with the onset of puberty. It is also a locally expansive condition. This disorder is thought to constitute 7% of all benign bone disorders (Coley 1968). Fibrous dysplasia is classified into three types:

1. Monostotic, where the bones usually affected are the femur, tibia, ribs, or facial bone. Of the facial bones, the maxilla and the mandible are commonly involved. Monostotic fibrous dysplasia accounts for 70% of fi-

brous dysplasias; when the temporal bone is involved, it is usually monostotic (Nager et al 1982).

2. In the polyostotic variety of fibrous dysplasia, the bones involved are frequently found in the lower limbs. When the facial bones are involved, the sphenoid is commonly involved. Polyostotic fibrous dysplasia accounts for 30% of cases; the craniofacial site is most common. In fibrous dysplasia, the temporal bone is involved in 18% of cases (Nager et al 1982).

3. The third variety is Albright's syndrome (Albright et al 1937; McCune 1936). McCune-Albright syndrome consists of the following features: polyostotic fibrous dysplasia that is unilaterally distributed, endocrinopathy (particularly hyperthyroidism), and cutaneous hyperpigmentation. This disorder primarily affects females who display precocious puberty.

Fibrous dysplasia typically erodes the cortical bone from within, normal bone being replaced by abnormal proliferative fibro-osseous tissue in the medullary cavity that, by erosion and expansion, transforms the cortex into a thin, weak shell. The remodeled bone is immature and structurally weak.

## Histopathology of Fibrous Dysplasia

Histologically, the fibrous dysplasia appears heterogeneous, with interspersed regions of bone and abnormal soft tissue. The soft tissue is filled with collagen, with intermediate areas of fibroblasts arranged in a whorl-like pattern. The bony areas demonstrate irregularly shaped immature trabeculae resembling coarse woven fiber rather than bone (Lambert and Brackmann 1984). The lack of osteoblastic rimming is conspicuous.

## Clinical Features of Fibrous Dysplasia

Stenosis of the external auditory canal, progressive hearing loss, and postauricular bony swelling are the predominant presenting features of temporal bone dysplasia. As the external auditory canal becomes gradually occluded, entrapment of epithelial debris occurs. This in turn leads to otorrhea and infection. A cholesteatoma of the external auditory canal can occur. Interestingly, the otic capsule is usually spared by the primary disease process. Usually any hearing loss that is present is conductive. Sensorineural hearing loss can also occur, but this is usually secondary to cholesteatoma or stenosis of the internal auditory canal. Facial nerve dysfunction is not a common manifestation of this disease.

## Radiological Imaging of Fibrous Dysplasia

Typical radiographic features on plain conventional x-rays for type 1, the sclerotic variety, include a homogeneous radiodensity accompanied by expansion of surrounding bone. The mass appears to have a typical ground glass appearance. In type 2, the pagetoid type areas of lucency surrounded by irregular scerosis is seen. In type 3, a cystic pattern is seen, as well as an ovoid radiolucency with a sclerotic border.

CT scanning is the imaging modality of choice for this disorder. All the anatomical areas of the temporal bone that have been compromised by the disease can be clearly demonstrated. The entire anatomical boundaries of the temporal bone in the coronal and axial plane also can be clearly demonstrated. The typical appearance of the fibrous dysplasia lesion can help identify the nature of the lesion. If doubt arises, a biopsy of the lesion to obtain a histopathological diagnosis may be necessary.

## Treatment of Fibrous Dysplasia

Currently, there is no specific medical treatment for this condition. Surgery is directed at maintaining a patent and wide external auditory canal. Restenosis of the external canal is common. Radical resection is not recommended; it can be quite hazardous because landmarks become obliterated and the disease process is quite vascular. Radical resection is also not feasible at times because of the extension of the disease. Furthermore, radical resection is not warranted in this benign condition.

Should a cranial nerve be compromised by the lesion, surgery is directed at decompressing the cranial nerve. Sarcomatous degeneration of fibrous dysplasia has been reported, although its incidence is very rare. It has been reported that there is a 0.4% incidence in monostotic and polyostotic fibrous dysplasia. The incidence rises (Lambert and Brackman, 1984) to 4.0% in the Albright's syndrome.

## REFERENCES

Adair Dighton CA. Four generations of blue sclerotics. *Ophthalmoscope.* 1912;10: 188–189.

Albright F, Butler A, Hampton A, Smith P. Syndrome characterized by osteitis fibrosa disseminata: Areas of pigmentation and endocrine dysfunction with precocious puberty in females. *NEJM.* 1937;216:727–746.

Armstrong BW. Stapes surgery in patients with osteogenesis imperfecta. *Ann Otol, Rhinol Laryngol.* 1984;93:634–636.

Arslan M, Ricci V. Histochemical investigation of otosclerosis with special regard to collagen disease. *J Laryngol Otol.* 1963;77:365–373.

Avioli LV. Paget's disease: State of the art. *Clin Thera.* 1987;9:567–576.

Berger G, Hawke M, Johnson A, Proops D. Histopathology of the temporal bone in osteogenesis imperfecta congenital: Report of five cases. *Laryngoscope.* 1986;95: 193–198.

Bergstrom LV. Osteogenesis imperfecta: otologic and maxillofacial aspects. *Laryngoscope.* 1977;87(suppl 6):1–42.

Bollerslev J, Andersen PE. Radiological, biochemical and hereditary evidence of two types of autosomal dominant osteopetrosis. *Bone.* 1988;9:7–13.

Bollerslev J, Grontved A, Andersen PE. Autosomal dominant osteopetrosis: An otoneurological investigation of the two radiological types. *Laryngoscope.* 1988; 98:411–413.

Bronson E. On fragilitus ossium and its association with blue sclerotics and otosclerosis. *Edinburgh Med J.* 1917;18:240–274.

Brosnan M, Burns H, Jahn AF, Hawk M. Surgical histopathology of the stapes in osteogenesis imperfecta tarda. *Arch Otolaryngol.* 1977;103:294–298.

Chevance LG. On some histochemical aspcts of the otosclerotic focus, state and significance of the sulfhydryl groups. *Acta Otolaryngol.* 1964;58:175–182.

Clarke CRA, Harrison MJG. Neurological manifestations of Paget's disease. *J Neurolog Sci.* 1978;38:171–178.

Coley BL. Fibrous dysplasia of the bone: review of 24 cases. *Am J Med.* 1968;44: 421–429.

Collins DH. Paget's disease of bone: Incidence and subclinical forms. *Lancet.* 1956;2: 51–57.

Davies DG. Paget's disease of the temporal bone. *Acta Otolaryngol.* 1968;242(suppl): 1–47.

Davies DG. The temporal bone in Paget's disease. *J Laryngol Otol.* 1970;84:553–560.

De Rose J, Singer FR, Avaranides A. Response of Paget's disease to porcine and salmon calcitonins. *Am J Med.* 1974;56:858–866.

Detheridge FM, Guyer PB, Barker DJP. European distribution of Paget's disease of the bone. *Brit Med J.* 1982;285:1005–1008.

Dort JC, Pollack A, Fisch U. The fallopian canal and the facial nerve in sclerosteosis of the temporal bone: A histopathologic study. *Am J Otolaryngol.* 1990;11(5):320–325.

Elias EG, Evans JT. Mithramycin in the treatment of Paget's disease of bone. *J Bone Joint Surg.* 1972;54:1730–1736.

Freeman DA. Southwestern internal medicine conference: Paget's disease of the bone. *Am J Med Sci.* 1988;295:144–158.

Gagel RF, Logan C, Mallette LE. Treatment of Paget's disease of bone with salmon calcitonin nasal spray. *JAGS.* 1988;36:1011–1014.

Garretsen AJ, Cremers CW, Huygen PL. Hearing loss (in nonoperated ears) in relation to age in osteogenesis imperfecta type I. *Ann Otol, Rhinol Laryngol.* 1997; 106:575–582.

Garretsen JTM, Cremers WRJ. Ear surgery in osteogenesis imperfecta. *Arch Otolaryngol.* 1990;116:317–323.

Gutman AB, Kasabach H. Paget's disease (osteitis deformans): Analysis of 116 cases. *Am J Med Sci.* 1936;191:361–380.

Haddad JG, Birge SJ, Avioli LV. Effect of prolonged thyrocalcitonin administration on Paget's disease of bone. *NEJM.* 1970;285:549–555.

Hammersma H. Osteopetrosis (marble bone disease) of the temporal bone. *Laryngoscope.* 1970;80:1518–1539.

Holdsworth CE, Endahl GL, Soifer N, Richardson KE, Eyring EJ. Comparative biochemical study of otosclerosis and osteogenesis imperfecta. *Arch Otolaryngol.* 1973;98:336–339.

Johnsson LG, Hawkins JE, Rousse RC, Linthicum FH. Cochlear and otoconial abnormalities in capsular otosclerosis and hydrops. *Ann Otol, Rhinol Laryngol.* 1982; 97(suppl):3–15.

Johnston CC Jr, Lavy N, Lord T, Vellios F, Merritt AD, Deiss WP Jr. Osteopetroses: A clinical, genetic, metabolic and morphologic study of the dominantly inherited benign form. *Medicine.* 1968;47(2):149–167.

Khetarpal U, Schuknecht HF. In search of pathologic correlates for hearing loss and vertigo in Paget's disease: A clinical and histopathologic study of 26 temporal bones. *Ann Otol, Rhinol Laryngol.* 1990;99(suppl 145):1–16.

Kosoy J, Maddox HE. Surgical findings in Van der Hoeve's syndrome. *Arch Otolaryngol.* 1971;93:115–122.

Lambert PR, Brackmann DE. Fibrous dysplasia of the temporal bone: The use of computerized tomography. *Otolaryngol—Head Neck Surg.* 1984;92:461–467.

Lando M, Hoover LA, Finerman G. Stabilization of hearing loss in Paget's disease with calcitonin and etidronate. *Arch Otolaryngol.* 1988;114:891–894.

Lindsay JR, Lehman RH. Histopathology of the temporal bone in advanced Paget's disease. *Laryngoscope.* 1969;79:213–227.

Lindsay JR, Perlman HB. Paget's disease and deafness. *Arch Otolaryngol.* 1936;23: 581–587.

Lindsay JR, Suga F. Paget's disease and sensorineural deafness: temporal bone histopathology of Paget's disease. *Laryngoscope.* 1976;86:1029–1042.

Marini JC. Osteogenesis imperfecta comprehensive management. *Adv Ped.* 1988;35: 391–426.

McCune DJ. Osteitis fibrosa cystica: The case of a nine-year-old girl who also exhibits precocious puberty, multiple pigmentation of the kin and hyperthyroidism. *Am J Dis Childhood.* 1936;52:745–748.

Mills BG, Singer FR. Nuclear inclusions in Paget's disease of bone. *Science.* 1976;194: 201–203.

Miyamoto RT, House WF, Brackmann DE. Neurotologic manifestations of the osteopetroses. *Arch Otolaryngol.* 1980;106:210–214.

Nager GT. Paget's disease of the temporal bone. *Ann Otolaryngol, Rhinol Laryngol.* 1975;84:(suppl 22):1–32.

Nager GT, Kennedy DW, Kopstein E. Fibrous dysplasia: a review of the disease and its manifestations in the temporal bone. *Ann Otol, Rhinol Laryngol.* 1982;91(suppl 91):1–52.

Paterson CR, Monk EA, McAllion SJ. How common is hearing impairment in osteogenesis imperfecta? *J Laryngol Otol.* 2001;6:280–282.

Pederson U. Hearing loss in patients with osteogenesis imperfecta. *Scand Audiol.* 1982;99:451–458.

Pedersen U. Osteogenesis imperfecta: Clinical features, hearing loss and stapedectomy. *Acta Otolaryngol Supplementum.* 1985;415:1–36.

Pedersen U, Elbrond O. Stapedectomy in osteogenesis imperfecta. *ORL J Otorhinolaryngol Relat Spec.* 1983;45: 330–337.

Pedersen U, Melsen F, Elbrond O, Charles P. Histopathology of the stapes in osteogenesis imperfecta. *J Otol Laryngol.* 1985;99:451–458.

Proops D, Bayley D, Hawke M. Paget's disease and the temporal bone: A clinical and histopathological review of six temporal bones. *J Otolaryngol.* 1985;14:20–29.

Quisiling RW, Moore GR, Jahrsdoerfer RA, Cantrell RW. Osteogenesis imperfecta: A study of 160 family members. *Arch Otolaryngol.* 1979;105:207–211.

Reginster JY, Albert A, Franchimont P. Salmon calcitonin spray in Paget's disease of bone: Preliminary results in five patients. *Calcif Tissue Int.* 1985;37:577–580.

Russell RGG, Fleisch H. Pyrophosphate and diphosphonates in skeletal metabolism. *Clin Orthoped.* 1975;108:241–263.

Ryan WG, Schwartz TB, Fordham EW. Mithramycin and long remission of Paget's disease of bone. *Ann Int Med.* 1980;92:129–130.

Shai F, Baker RK, Wallach S. The clinical and metabolic effects of porcine calcitonin on Paget's disease of bone. *J Clin Invest.* 1971;50:1927–1940.

Shapiro JR, Pikus A, Weiss G, Rowe DW. Hearing and middle ear function in osteogenesis imperfecta. *JAMA.* 1982;247:2120–2126.

Shea JJ, Postma DS. Findings and long-term surgical results in the hearing loss of osteogenesis imperfecta. *Arch Otolaryngol.* 1982;108:467–470.

Sillence DO, Senn A, Danks DM. Genetic heterogeneity in osteogenesis imperfecta. *J Med Genet.* 1979;16:101–116.

Smith R, Russell RGG, Bishop M. Diphosphonates and Paget's disease of bone. *Lancet.* 1971;1:945–947.

Sparrow NJ, Duval AJ. Hearing loss and Paget's disease. *J Laryngol Otol.* 1967; 81:601–611.

Stewart EJ, O'Reilly BF. A clinical and audiological investigation of osteogenesis imperfecta. *Clin Otolaryngol.* 1989;14:509–514.

Swartz JD, Harnsberger HR. The otic capsule and otodystrophies. In: *Imaging of the Temporal Bone.* 2nd ed. New York: Thieme; 1992:192–246.

Uppal HS, D'Souza AR, Proops DW. Osseointegration in Paget's disease: The bone anchored hearing aid in the rehabilitation of pagetic deafness. *J Laryngol Otol.* 2001;115:903–906.

Van der Hoeve J, de Kleyn A. Blau sclera knochenkruchig-keit und Schwerhorig-Keit. *Arch Ophthalmologie.* 1918;95:81–93.

Walker DG. Osteopetrosis cured by temporary parabiosis. *Science.* 1973;180:875.

Walker DG. Bone resorption restored in osteopetrotic mice by transplants of normal bone marrow and spleen cells. *Science.* 1975a;190:784–785.

Walker DG. Control of bone resorption by hematopoietic tissue: the induction and reversal of congenital osteopetrosis in mice through use of bone marrow and splenic transplants. *J Exper Med.* 1975b;142:651–653.

*Chapter 18*

# The Biomechanics of Stapes Replacement

In humans, the rigidity of the annular ligament represents almost 90% of the impedance of the middle ear, especially at low frequencies (Huttenbrink 2003). This annular ligament therefore dominates the transmission of sound at speech frequencies in the normal middle ear in humans. The collagen fibers of the annular ligament determine the amplitude with which the stapedial footplate will vibrate in response to low-frequency acoustic stimulation. The sound pressure at the entrance of the cochlea is directly proportional to the volume velocity of the stapes footplate, which in turn corresponds to the volume of the liquid that is displaced by the vibration of the stapes footplate. The output of the middle ear can be quantified by the "volume velocity" of the stapes footplate. Volume velocity can be defined as the product of stapes linear velocity and the area of the stapes footplate (Rosowski and Merchant 1995).

The stapes footplate has an area of approximately 3.2 mm$^2$. This exerts vibrations with amplitudes of only a few nanometers for displacement of a large amount of fluid to transmit sound pressure into the cochlea at physiologic sound pressures. Therefore, following stapedotomy, the effective vibrating area is reduced to the area where the prosthesis has been inserted, reducing in turn the volume velocity. A stapes prosthesis, with its smaller contact area (32 mm$^2$ area of footplate vs. 0.12 mm$^2$ area of fenestra in a 0.4 mm$^2$ stapes prosthesis), can vibrate with much larger amplitude at equivalent sound pressures. Compensation takes place because the increased linear velocity of the smaller piston compensates for the decrease in the surface area.

## HOW THE BIOMECHANICAL ACTIVITY OF THE MIDDLE EAR IS STUDIED

The biomechanical activity of the middle ear is studied in animal models, human cadaveric temporal bones, and mathematical models. Modern tools like laser Doppler vibrometry have provided better insight into the acoustic effects of stapedectomy/stapedotomy in humans. Mathematical models like the finite element model (FEM) and the simple lumped element model have a disadvantage in that any single incorrect parameter can distort a result.

## APPLICATION OF BIOMECHANICS ON THE SEAL OF THE FENESTRA

The interface between the piston and the edge of the fenestra is considered to simulate the stiffness of the annular ligament (Causse 1989). The seal, in addition to transmitting pressure changes in a uniform manner in all directions in the vestibule, stabilizes the piston against changes in atmospheric pressure (Huttenbrink 2003). The vibrating (and therefore the energy transferring) area of the stapes prosthesis, is not limited to the diameter of the prosthesis. It will also include the area of the surrounding connective seal, which, being larger than the diameter of the piston, gives good results in hearing (Smyth and Hassard 1978).

## APPLICATION OF PRESERVATION OF THE STAPES TENDON IN STAPES REPLACEMENT

Silverstein and colleagues (1998) found that preservation of the stapes tendon reduced incus erosion because the blood supply to the lenticular process was kept intact. Furthermore, they postulated that there was a more physiologic transmission for high sound pressure levels and a reduction in the discomfort in a noisy environment because of the preservation of the acoustic reflex.

In a normal ear, the pull of the stapes muscle rotates the footplate around its transverse axis and thus stretches the annular ligament, causing an increase in the tension of the collagen fibers of the annular ligament. This in turn causes a shift of the resonance to the higher frequencies (Huttenbrink 1995). The acoustic reflex induces a decrease of larger movements of the footplate and low-frequency transmission but an improved transmission of the more harmful higher frequencies of noise. Thus, it would seem that the preservation of the stapes muscle in stapedotomy does not serve the purpose for which it was intended.

Following stapedotomy with preservation of the stapedius muscle, a contraction of the stapedius muscle could be registered as a change in impedance of the tympanic membrane. Impedance change of the fenestral seal between the piston and the vestibule, however, cannot be estimated. At this time it is unclear what the other factors are that contribute to the pleasant hearing experienced by patients who have undergone stapedotomy and have had the stapedius muscle preserved (Huttenbrink 2003).

## CORRECT CRIMPING OF THE STAPES PISTON AROUND THE MALLEUS AND INCUS

### Malleovestibulopexy

Angulation of the stapes prosthesis will be evident where the incus has been bypassed and the prosthesis is crimped around the malleus, especially if the fenestra is placed in the posterior aspect of the footplate. Should the prosthesis in this case touch the surrounding bone, this would result in an attenuation of the vibration, with resulting decrease in sound transmission (Hausler 2000). The malleus handle is located anteriorly to the oval window and can thus cause the prosthesis to come in contact with bony edges of the fenestra that in turn will dampen its vibrations. Additionally, loose coupling of the prosthesis to the malleus handle could further contribute to dampening of sound transmission. Thus, the overall hearing result will be inferior under these circumstances. For better hearing results, the prosthesis should be angled and should be crimped firmly at the malleus handle. This will prevent any tilting movement. Hearing results can be further improved by tightening the wire loop around the handle of the malleus.

## Prosthesis from the Incus to the Fenestra

Firm attachment of the prosthesis to the long process of the incus is the dominant factor for effective energy transmission. Huttenbrink (2003) believed that the choice of material is irrelevant as long as the prosthesis is firmly anchored. A finite element model analysis demonstrated that loose coupling results in additional lateral ineffective vibrations (Blayney, Williams, and Rice 1997; Williams, Blayney, and Lesser 1995).

Loosening of the attachment because of the erosion of the incus is the most common cause for a postoperative air-bone gap. One school of thought was that tight crimping of the prosthesis caused a reduction in blood supply (Schimanski 1997). Another postulate was that there is increased force at the wire loop with atmospheric pressure-induced movements of the incus if the prosthesis is tightly fastened in connective tissue in the oval window niche (Schimanski 1998).

The lenticular process of the incus is displaced only a few micrometers at atmospheric variations because the malleus incus joint attenuates the movements of the tympanic membrane (Huttenbrink 1988). These displacements are too small to build up a pressure that would cause bone resorption. The cause of incus resorption is not pressure-induced changes; instead, a foreign body reaction is considered likely (Huttenbrink 2003).

## DOES THE DIAMETER OF THE STAPES PROSTHESIS (PISTONS) AFFECT THE HEARING RESULT?

The diameter of the stapes prosthesis does indeed influence the hearing result. Merchant and Rosowski (2003) and Goode (2003) reported that larger area pistons perform better than smaller area pistons, particularly at frequencies below 1.5 kHz. Merchant and Rosowski (2003) believed that there is no single optimum piston diameter; instead, there is a continuum where larger piston diameters give better hearing results They stated that the smaller the area of the prosthesis, the greater the air-bone gap. Goode and Hato (2000) measured round window velocity in experimental temporal bones with stapes prostheses of varying diameter. Round pistons of 0.4 mm diameter and 0.8 mm diameter and an oval 1.6 x 0.8 mm piston were used while keeping all of the other parameters unchanged. The results showed significant differences between different piston diameters. The pistons with the larger diameters produced the larger round window velocities.

## Behavior of Stapes Prostheses When Subjected to Atmospheric Variations

The ear behaves like a pressure receptor by transmitting acoustic sound pressure to the inner ear. When performing tympanometry, the pressure changes of ± 400 mm $H_2O$ on the tympanic membrane and the malleus are displaced inward and outward by a distance of up to 1 mm. In the normal ossicular chain, these forces cause a gliding movement at the malleus incus joint. These gliding movements force the incus either upward or downward, as the situation may be. Because of this change of the outward-outward movement of the malleus to a perpendicular movement at the lenticular process, the stapes and the inner ear are uncoupled from the extensive displacements of the tympanic membrane at ambient air pressures. The maximum movement of the stapes and the footplate never exceeds 10 to 30 μm regardless of the pressure in the external ear canal (Huttenbrink 1988). This protective mechanism occurs because of the annular ligament. In stapedotomy, this protective mechanism is now absent, and the prosthesis can move almost unrestrictedly in the vestibule. Furthermore, larger displacements of the prosthesis can be expected if the gliding movements of the malleus and incus are impaired. Thus, it can be seen that a short piston can be displaced from the fenestra by simple sneezing or by a Valsalva maneuver and can then result in a postoperative conductive hearing loss. On the other hand, a longer piston can impale the structures of the vestibule, which in turn can result in vertigo and even hearing loss. Therefore, the fenestra in which the piston is to be inserted should be placed in the posterior part of the footplate.

Huttenbrink (2003) proposed that the insertion length of the piston should be 0.5 mm into the fenestra. This will prevent displacement of the prosthesis from the fenestra and will also prevent it from damaging either the utricle or the saccule.

The seal should also mature and heal completely. Therefore, air travel should not be permitted until the seal of the fenestra has matured and healed completely. This takes approximately 2 to 3 weeks (Harrill, Jenkins, and Coker 1996). This is because even in modern passenger jets flying at 41,00 feet the cabin pressure differential relative to sea level is 2000 mm $H_2O$. This can induce excessive displacements of the tympanic membrane even with repeated multiple tubal openings (Syms 1991).

Tympanometry with simultaneous electronystagmography recording is performed on those patients who are candidates for stapedotomy while being subjected to excessive pressure variants. If no vertigo or pathologic eye movements are evoked with pressures of 400 mm $H_2O$, then such patients can safely undergo stapedotomy. This has been confirmed by several reports where stapedotomy has been performed on military pilots (Katzav, Lippy, and Shamiss 1996; Rayman 1972; Thiringer and Arriaga 1998).

Another factor that should be considered in such patients is that the tympanic membrane should be in good health. Divers with an atrophic tympanic membrane run the risk of rupturing their tympanic membranes if they are atrophic.

# REFERENCES

Blayney AW, Williams KR, Rice HJ. A dynamic and harmonic damped finite element analysis model of stapedotomy. *Acta Otolaryngologica*. 1997;117:269–273.

Causse JB. The twenty fine points of otosclerosis surgery. *Am J Otolaryngol*. 1989; 10:75–77.

Goode RL. Invited comment on Biomechanics of stapesplasty. *Otol Neurotol*. 2003; 24:557–559.

Goode RL, Hato N. A temporal bone model of stapedotomy for otosclerosis. *Otolaryngol Head Neck Surg*. 2000;123:86–87.

Harrill WG, Jenkins HA, Coker NJ. Barotrauma after stapes surgery: a survey of recommended restrictions and clinical experiences. *Am J Otolaryngol*. 1996;17:835–846.

Hausler R. Advances in stapes surgery (in German). *Laryngol Rhinol Otol*. 2000;79 (suppl 2):95–139.

Huttenbrink KB. The mechanics of the middle ear at static air pressure. *Acta Otolaryngol*. 1988;451(suppl):1–36.

Huttenbrink KB. The function of the ossicular chain and of the muscles of the middle ear (in German). *Euro Arch Otorhinolaryngol*. 1995 (suppl 1):1–52.

Huttenbrink KB. Biomechanics of stapesplasty: a review. *Otol Neurotol*. 2003;24: 548–557.

Katzav J, Lippy WH, Shamiss A. Stapedectomy in combat pilots. *Am J Otolaryngol*. 1996:17:847–849.

Merchant SN, Rosowski JJ. Invited comment on Biomechanics of stapesplasty. *Otol Neurotol*. 2003;24:557–559.

Rayman RB. Stapedectomy: a threat to flying safety? *Aerospace Med*. 1972;43:545–550.

Rosowski JJ, Merchant SN. Mechanical and acoustic analysis of middle ear reconstruction. *Am J Otolaryngol*. 1995;16:486–497.

Schimanski G. Erosion and necrosis of the long process of the incus after otosclerosis surgery. (in German). *HNO*. 1997;45:682–689.

Schimanski G. Stapes surgery in otosclerosis (in German). *HNO*. 1998;46:289–295.

Silverstein H, Hester O, Rosenberg S, Deems D. Preservation of the stapes tendon in laser stapes surgery. *Laryngoscope*. 1998;108:1453–1458.

Smyth GDL, Hassard TH. Eighteen years experience in stapedectomy: the case for the small fenestra operation. *Ann Otol Rhinol Laryngol*. 1978;87(suppl):3–36.

Syms CA. Flying after otologic surgery. *Am J Otol*. 1991;12:162.

Thiringer JK, Arriaga MA. Stapedectomy in military air crew. *Otolaryngol Head Neck Surg*. 1998;118:9–14.

Williams KR, Blayney AW, Lesser TM. A three dimensional finite element analysis of the natural frequencies of vibration of a stapes prosthesis replacement reconstruction of the middle ear. *Clin Otolaryngol*. 1995;20:36–44.

# Appendix: Quiz

1. At what age is clinical otosclerosis commonly first noticed?
   A. 20 to 30 years
   B. 30 to 40 years
   C. 40 to 50 years

2. Is there a real racial predisposition?
   A. Yes
   B. No

3. Caucasians are more predisposed to developing otosclerosis.
   A. True
   B. False

4. According to the available literature on otosclerosis, men are more affected than women.
   A. True
   B. False

5. Otosclerosis can present as
   A. Conductive hearing loss
   B. Sensorineural hearing loss
   C. Mixed hearing loss
   D. No symptoms
   E. All of the above

6. Histologic otosclerosis is a disease process that is often discovered postmortem as an incidental finding.
   A. True
   B. False

7. Histologic otosclerosis is a disease process without clinical findings or manifestations.
   A. True
   B. False

8. Otosclerosis affects only the otic capsule and ossicles of the temporal bones.
   A. True
   B. False

9. The most common location of the otosclerotic focus is the round window.
   A. True
   B. False

10. Otosclerosis is a localized bone remodeling process.
    A. True
    B. False

11. Otosclerosis has two phases: an active phase and a sclerotic (inactive) phase.
    A. True
    B. False

**12.** Otosclerosis presents in a familial (hereditary) and sporadic pattern.
 **A.** True
 **B.** False

**13.** Genetic (familial, hereditary) otosclerosis is thought to be present as an autosomal dominant transmission with incomplete penetration.
 **A.** True
 **B.** False

**14.** Recently the paramyxovirus (measles virus) has been implicated as a cause of otosclerosis.
 **A.** True
 **B.** False

**15.** The paramyxovirus infects the following:
 **A.** Fissula ante fenestram
 **B.** Fossula ante fenestram
 **C.** Globuli interossei
 **D.** Malleus

**16.** Otosclerosis typically presents as a low-frequency conductive hearing loss in the initial stages.
 **A.** True
 **B.** False

**17.** The typical pattern of cochlear otosclerosis is the "cookie bite" pattern, where the greatest degree of hearing loss is in the mid-frequency hearing range.
 **A.** True
 **B.** False

**18.** Is Carhart's notch typical of otosclerosis?
 **A.** Yes
 **B.** No

**19.** Middle ear aeration is not affected in otosclerosis.
 **A.** True
 **B.** False

**20.** In impedance audiometry, static compliance values less than 0.3 cc are considered to be in keeping with a diagnosis of otosclerosis.
 **A.** True
 **B.** False

**21.** There is evidence of an association between an increase in stapedial otosclerosis and low sodium fluoride levels in water.
 **A.** True
 **B.** False

**22.** Sodium fluoride should be administered under the following circumstances:
 **A.** Surgically confirmed otosclerosis with sensorineural hearing loss disproportionate to age
 **B.** A positive Schwartze's sign
 **C.** Patients who have a sensorineural hearing loss with a family history of otosclerosis

D. Patients who have otosclerosis and vestibular symptoms
E. All of the above
F. None of the above

23. An alternative to sodium fluoride therapy is
A. Biphosphonates
B. Cytokine inhibitors
C. Methotrexate
D. Cisplatin

24. CT scanning is the imaging modality of choice to make a diagnosis of otosclerosis.
A. True
B. False

25. CT scanning is of some use in diagnosing cochlear otosclerosis.
A. True
B. False

26. CT densitometry is a quantitative, objective way of evaluating involvement of the cochlear capsule.
A. True
B. False

27. MRI is indicated in the postoperative period to evaluate the status of the prosthesis.
A. True
B. False

28. Hearing aids should be offered as a viable alternative to patients who suffer from otosclerosis.
A. True
B. False

29. Paracusis of Willis is a phenomenon in which the person suffering from otosclerosis experiences an apparent improvement in hearing in the midst of ambient sound.
A. True
B. False

30. The carbon dioxide laser, but for its cumbersome micromanipulator system, is excellent for stapedectomy.
A. True
B. False

31. Currently, there is no single ideal laser for stapedectomy.
A. True
B. False

32. Lasers are ideal tools for revision stapedectomy.
A. True
B. False

33. Stapedectomy is far superior to stapedotomy.
A. True
B. False

34. Stapedotomy is apparently better than partial stapedectomy.
    A. True
    B. False

35. A patient who presents with hydrops and otosclerosis can undergo surgery as soon as the symptoms of hydrops are controlled.
    A. True
    B. False

36. Signs and symptoms of a perilymph fistula include
    A. Fluctuating hearing loss
    B. Tinnitus
    C. Unconsciousness
    D. Vertigo
    E. Diarrhea
    F. All of the above
    G. A, B, and D
    H. C and D

37. Perilymph fistulae pose a real risk of meningitis.
    A. True
    B. False

38. Perilymph fistulae should be treated as surgical emergencies.
    A. True
    B. False

39. Untreated perilymph fistulae can result in permanent sensorineural hearing loss.
    A. True
    B. False

40. Ankylosis of the malleus is usually discovered during the course of stapedectomy.
    A. True
    B. False

41. Malleus ankylosis can be detected by pneumatic otoscopy and by observing the excursion of the tympanic membrane.
    A. True
    B. False

42. The second ear can be operated on as soon as the patient has recovered from the first stapedectomy.
    A. True
    B. False

43. Stapedectomy can be performed on the only hearing ear.
    A. Yes
    B. No

44. A positive Schwartze's sign indicates the following:
    A. Contraindication for surgery
    B. Active otosclerotic focus
    C. Possible cochlear otosclerosis
    D. All of the above

**45.** A cerebrospinal fluid gusher could be due to
    **A.** A patent cochlear aqueduct
    **B.** A defect in the fundus of the internal auditory meatus
    **C.** Traumatic rupture of the meninges
    **D.** All of the above
    **E.** A and B

**46.** Far advanced otosclerosis is a contraindication for stapedectomy.
    **A.** True
    **B.** False

**47.** There is a distinct learning curve among residents performing stapedectomy.
    **A.** True
    **B.** False

**48.** Causes of conductive hearing loss following stapedectomy include
    **A.** Necrosis of the long process of the incus
    **B.** Migration of the prosthesis
    **C.** Adhesions
    **D.** Regrowth of the otosclerotic focus
    **E.** Slipped prosthesis
    **F.** Ankylosis of the head of the malleus
    **G.** All of the above
    **H.** A, B, and D

**49.** Gelfoam is a suitable oval window seal following stapedectomy.
    **A.** True
    **B.** False

**50.** Stapedectomy can be performed in athletes who run the risk of possible trauma to the head.
    **A.** True
    **B.** False

**51.** Manage the floating footplate by
    **A.** Terminating the procedure
    **B.** Removing the footplate by a previously created pothole
    **C.** Placing the prosthesis on top of the footplate
    **D.** Tipping the footplate into the vestibule by using gentle suction
    **E.** All of the above
    **F.** A, B, and C

**52.** Congenital fixation of the footplate is associated with a perilymph gusher.
    **A.** True
    **B.** False

**53.** Heavier prostheses usually give better hearing results.
    **A.** True
    **B.** False

**54.** The most common cause of failure of stapedectomy is
    **A.** Migration of the prosthesis
    **B.** Incus resorption osteitis

C. Regrowth of new bone at the site of the fenestra
D. Perilymph fistula
E. Tympanic membrane perforation

55. Persistent stapedial artery is a contraindication for stapedectomy.
   A. True
   B. False

56. Obliteration of the oval window usually means
   A. Surgery should be abandoned.
   B. Regrowth of new bone is common.
   C. Perilymph fistula is common.
   D. The prosthesis should be a little longer.
   E. A larger fenestra should be created.
   F. All of the above
   G. A, B, and C
   H. B, D, and E

57. Lasers are the best tool to create a fenestra when dealing with obliterative otosclerosis.
   A. True
   B. False

58. A reparative granuloma must
   A. Be promptly removed with lasers
   B. Be treated with steroids only
   C. Be passively observed
   D. Be treated with antibiotics

59. Endolymphatic hydrops can develop poststapedectomy even when hydrops was not present previously.
   A. True
   B. False

60. Stapedectomy can be performed in those patients who have a conductive hearing loss and who suffer from
   A. Paget's disease of the bone
   B. Osteopetrosis
   C. Osteogenesis imperfecta
   D. Fibrous dysplasia

61. Which procedure is associated with the fewest complications?
   A. Total stapedectomy
   B. Partial stapedectomy
   C. Small fenestra stapedectomy

62. When a floating footplate is encountered, the best thing to do is
   A. Abandon surgery
   B. Remove the footplate and opt for total stapedectomy
   C. Carry on with stapedectomy
   D. Ignore it

63. When a ptotic facial nerve that completely covers the oval window is encountered, one should

    A. Decompress the facial nerve
    B. Reroute the facial nerve
    C. Proceed with stapedectomy
    D. Abandon surgery

64. A tissue seal is preferred to a fat or Gelfoam seal.
    A. True
    B. False

65. Hearing aids should always be included as a treatment option for otosclerosis.
    A. True
    B. False

66. Hearing aids are covered by most insurance companies in the United States.
    A. True
    B. False

67. There is no learning curve when learning how to do a stapedectomy (especially during residency) provided that the teaching program is exceptional.
    A. True
    B. False

68. Total obliteration of the round window is rare.
    A. True
    B. False

69. Elderly patients should be denied a stapedectomy because of their age.
    A. True
    B. False

70. Otosclerosis affects all the bones of the human body.
    A. True
    B. False

## ANSWER KEY

1. A

2. A

3. A

4. B

5. E

6. A

7. A

8. A

9. B; the oval window is the most common site.

10. A

11. A

12. A

13. A

14. A

15. C

16. A

17. A

18. A; although it is typical of otosclerosis, it can occur in any condition that reduces the vibration of the stapes footplate.

19. A

20. A

21. A

22. E

23. A

24. B

25. A

26. A

27. B

28. A

29. A

30. A

31. A

32. A

33. B

34. A. However, many authors agree that there is a definite bias toward stapedotomy in the literature and claim that results in hearing of both techniques are in fact the same. Complications such as perilymph fistulae are less common with stapedotomy.

35. B; the patient must be free from symptoms of hydrops for a minimum period of 6 months.

36. G

37. A

38. A

39. A

40. A

**41.** A

**42.** B

**43.** B; it is an absolute contraindication.

**44.** D

**45.** E

**46.** B

**47.** A

**48.** G

**49.** B

**50.** B

**51.** F

**52.** A

**53.** A

**54.** A

**55.** B

**56.** H

**57.** A

**58.** A

**59.** A

**60.** C

**61.** C

**62.** A

**63.** D

**64.** A

**65.** A

**66.** B

**67.** B

**68.** A

**69.** B

**70.** B

# Index